In Clinical Practice

Taking a practical approach to clinical medicine, this series of smaller reference books is designed for the trainee physician, primary care physician, nurse practitioner and other general medical professionals to understand each topic covered. The coverage is comprehensive but concise and is designed to act as a primary reference tool for subjects across the field of medicine.

Nick A. Aresti
Matthew Barry
Mark (J.M.H.) Paterson
Manoj Ramachandran
Editors

Paediatric Orthopaedic Trauma in Clinical Practice

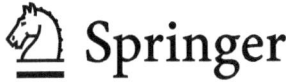 Springer

Editors

Nick A. Aresti
Percivall Pott Rotation
London
UK

Mark (J.M.H.) Paterson
The Royal London Hospital
London
UK

Matthew Barry
The Royal London Hospital
London
UK

Manoj Ramachandran
The Royal London Hospital
London
UK

ISSN 2199-6652   ISSN 2199-6660   (electronic)
In Clinical Practice
ISBN 978-1-4471-6755-6   ISBN 978-1-4471-6756-3   (eBook)
DOI 10.1007/978-1-4471-6756-3

Library of Congress Control Number: 2015956784

Springer London Heidelberg New York Dordrecht

Printed on acid-free paper

Springer-Verlag London Ltd. is part of Springer Science+Business Media (www.springer.com)

This book is in loving memory of Mark (J.M.H.) Paterson, our dedicated colleague and trusted friend

Dedicated to my wonderful wife-to-be, Stephanie
Nick A. Aresti

For Caroline and my children Max, Fran, Felix and Joe
Matthew Barry

As always, for my wife, Joanna, and my daughters Isabel and Mia
Manoj Ramachandran

Mark (J.M.H.) Paterson (1954–2013)

Mark (J.M.H.) Paterson was a key figure in developing children's orthopaedic services in East London. He was born in Hong Kong to a family with a history of missionary service. Mark followed his father in studying medicine at the Middlesex Hospital Medical School, graduating in 1977. After house jobs in Norwich, he spent a year working as a Medical Officer in Papua New Guinea where he found himself undertaking varied medical, surgical and even gynaecological work. He then returned to UK training with junior posts in and around the Southeast, and in 1986 was appointed Senior Registrar on the London Hospital training programme. This provided him with opportunity to work at the Royal London and Royal National Orthopaedic Hospitals, and he travelled abroad to gain experience in San Diego and Connecticut. With this experience behind him, he was appointed to the staff of the then London Hospital in 1990 to work initially with Brian Roper in building the services for children. Following Brian Roper's retirement and the ever-increasing demand, Mark's role in the department gradually evolved from a consultant with a special interest in children's orthopaedics to a full-time children's practice.

With the increased centralisation of children's services he soon required additional colleagues and during his career transformed a part-time commitment by one consultant to a department of four children's orthopaedic surgeons. Mark's particular forte was the difficult area of neuromuscular orthopaedics and notably cerebral palsy where his gentle manner, endless patience and understanding endeared him to his patients, their parents and his colleagues. Despite his hectic work schedule he was an examiner for the FRCS (Orth) for five years and assessor of examiners for a further year. He also examined for the European Board of Orthopaedics and Trauma and for the College of Surgeons in Hong Kong. Additionally he was involved with various surgical societies and President of the Orthopaedic Section of the Royal Society of Medicine 2006–2007. He believed passionately in providing healthcare for the underprivileged, and between 2009 and 2012 undertook six charitable missions to Albania where he was involved in the assessment and treatment of children with disability. Mark was an editor of the JBJS journal and also chaired their electronic publishing committee. He helped establish the EFORT/BESBJS Travelling Fellowships, which will continue in his memory. In January 2013, Mark retired from the NHS with the intention of continuing to provide children's services in the independent sector and participating in short-term projects in the third world. Sadly this was not to be due to the untimely intervention of neoplastic disease. He leaves his wife Sarah, whom he met as an undergraduate, and two sons Luke and Jamie. His ever-present, quiet, sensible and unstinting personality will be greatly missed by all of those whose lives he touched.

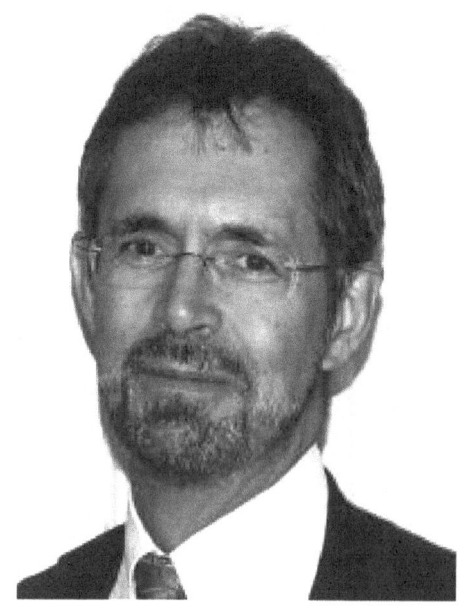

Introduction

It is vital that anyone training in orthopaedics is well versed in the art and practice of orthopaedic trauma. Paediatric orthopaedic trauma presents its own unique challenges, from the assessment of the injured child (and management of the parents and extended family) through to intervention with minimal complication and follow-up for long-term complications. The aim of this handbook is to cover all the major aspects of paediatric orthopaedic trauma and to ease the passage through examinations, such as the FRCS(Orth), and busy on-calls, where common children's fractures are frequently encountered.

Everything you need to know to gain confidence in paediatric orthopaedic trauma is right here in this book. Enjoy!

Manoj Ramachandran, MBBS (Hons),
MRCS, FRCS (Tr&Orth)
The Royal London Hospital,
London, UK

Contents

Contributors

Nick A. Aresti, MBBS, MRCS, PGCertMedEd, FHEA T&O SpR Percivall Pott Rotation, London, UK

Matthew Barry, MS, FRCS (Orth) Consultant Orthopaedic and Trauma Surgeon, Paediatric and Young Adult Orthopaedic Unit, The Royal London and The London Children's Hospitals, Barts Health NHS Trust, London, UK

Edward Britton, FRCS (Tr&Orth) T&O SpR Royal London Rotation, London, UK

Panteleimon Chan, MBBS, BSc (Hons), MRCS, MRCGP Davenport House Surgery, Harpenden, Hertfordshire, UK

Nima Heidari, MBBS, MSc, FRCS (Tr&Orth) Consultant Orthopaedic and Trauma Surgeon, The Royal London Limb Reconstruction Service, The Royal London and Barts and The London Children's Hospitals, Barts Health, London, UK

Thomas W. Hester, MBBS, BSc (Hons), MRCS T&O SpR South East Thames, London, UK

Keng Suan Khor, MBBS, BSc, (Hons), MRCS T&O SpR Percivall Pott Rotation, London, UK

Claudia Maizen, MD, FRCS (Orth) Consultant Orthopaedic and Trauma Surgeon, The Royal London and Barts and The London Children's Hospitals, Barts Health, London, UK

Alex Mulligan, MBBS, MRCS, MA (Cantab) T&O SpR Percivall Pott Rotation, London, UK

Mark (J.M.H.) Paterson, FRCS Paediatric and Young Adult Orthopaedic Unit, The Royal London and Barts and The London Children's Hospitals, Barts Health NHS Trust, London, UK

Anna C. Peek, FRCS (Tr&Orth) T&O SpR Percivall Pott Rotation, London, UK

Manoj Ramachandran, MBBS (Hons), MRCS, FRCS (Tr&Orth) Consultant Orthopaedic and Trauma Surgeon, Paediatric and Young Adult Orthopaedic Unit, The Royal London and Barts and The London Children's Hospitals, Barts Health NHS Trust, London, UK

John Stammers, MBBS, BSc (Hons), MRCS T&O SpR Royal London Rotation, London, UK

Joanna Thomas, MSc, FRCS (Tr&Orth) T&O SpR Royal London Rotation, London, UK

Kalpesh R. Vaghela, MBBS, BSc, MRCS, DipMedEd T&O SpR Percivall Pott Rotation, London, UK

Chapter 1
The Response to Injury in the Child & Bone Healing

Thomas W. Hester and Matthew Barry

1.1 Metabolic Response to Trauma in Children

The paediatric trauma patient differs in important ways from the adult, particularly with the nutritional requirements and protein catabolism. The response to trauma is classically described as two phases and this is largely the same for children. The initial ebb phase is characterised by decreased cardiac output, temperature, blood pressure and oxygen consumption. This is followed by the flow phase, with increased cardiac output, increased core temperature and elevated expression of catabolic hormones, leading to muscle breakdown.

The response to trauma begins in the immune system at the moment of injury. There is activation of macrophages and production of pro-inflammatory mediators in the injured tissue. In the microcirculation, activation of endothelial cells

T.W. Hester, MBBS, BSc (Hons), MRCS (✉)
T&O SpR South East Thames, London, UK
e-mail: thomashester@gmail.com

M. Barry, MS, FRCS (Orth)
Consultant Orthopaedic and Trauma Surgeon,
Paediatric and Young Adult Orthopaedic Unit,
The Royal London and Barts and The London Children's Hospitals,
Barts Health NHS Trust, London, UK

N.A. Aresti et al. (eds.), *Paediatric Orthopaedic Trauma in Clinical Practice*, In Clinical Practice,
DOI 10.1007/978-1-4471-6756-3_1,
© Springer-Verlag London Ltd. 2015

causes capillary leakage. These processes are potentiated by ischaemia, stimulating the cytokine system as a final common pathway resulting in the systemic inflammatory response.

This cascade consequently rapidly utilises glucose. Children have limited glycogen stores, increasing the need for gluco-neogenesis utilising, amongst other substrates, glucogenic amino acids (e.g. alanine and glutamine). Given children's protein stores are small, muscles are used as a source of pro-tein. Catabolism of diaphragmatic and intercostal muscles occurs within a week of injury.

Protein catabolism is activated primarily to protect the central nervous system, with the glucose being used by the brain as the main terminal oxidation site. This catabolic state and concomi-tant negative nitrogen balance may continue for weeks after acute injuries. With increasing severity of injury, there is an increase in the duration of catabolic states and this may adversely affect the rate of callus formation and fracture healing.

An optimal metabolic environment is needed for fracture healing, which in turn requires adequate protein and caloric intake. If in the event that oral feeding cannot be achieved, then nasogastric or total parentral nutrition should be considered.

Some major differences in children (compared to adults):

- Higher energy expenditure per kg of weight.
- Greater gut perfusion to absorb calories, leaving patients more vulnerable to mucosal ischaemia.
- Children do not increase energy expenditure in response to injury, instead shunting energy from growth (protein synthesis) while keeping total energy expenditure approx-imately the same.
- Higher rates of protein turnover.

1.2   Bone Healing in Children

This is commonly described in three phases:

- Inflammatory.
- Reparative.
- Remodelling.

1.2.1   Inflammatory

- Initial injury to the periosteum results in initiation of the repair process by release of growth factors, cytokines and prostaglandins.
- Coagulation and platelet activation stops blood loss and increases vascular permeability, allowing the passage of inflammatory cells, fibroblasts and stem cells into the fracture site.
- Neovascularisation is initiated by PDGF, VEGF and TGF β promoting osteoblast recruitment and activation.
- Initial local necrosis, due to disruption of the blood supply, further causes the release of growth factors, promoting mesenchymal cell differentiation.
- Organisation of the haematoma by fibroblastic cells resulting in a matrix rich in collagen I, III and V to support new woven bone.

1.2.2   Reparative

- Formation of woven bone forming the primary callus.
- This results from both endochondral ossification at the endosteal source and intramembranous ossification at the periosteum.
- Woven bone or primary callus is laid down in a haphazard manner, requiring large amounts to stabilize the fracture before the next phase can be entered.

1.2.3   Remodelling

- This is the longest phase and can last several years.
- The critical step between the reparative and remodelling phases is the establishment of an intact bony bridge between the fragments.
- Remodelling begins with the removal of mechanically unnecessary bone and ends in bone that is orientated to the lines of stress forming quality bone i.e. cancellous or cortical bone.

- Many factors are involved in the remodelling phase including Receptor activator of nuclear factor kappa-B (RANK) and Receptor activator of nuclear factor kappa-B ligand and (RANK-L) which are vital for differentiation of osteoclast progenitor cells.

1.3   Remodelling in the Injured Child

Three major factors have a bearing on the potential for remodelling:

- Skeletal age.
- Distance to the joint.
- Orientation to the joint.

There are slight differences in the characteristics of remodelling at the metaphysis and diaphysis:

1.3.1   Metaphysis

This is an active remodelling area in normal bone growth. It is the area where the quantity of woven bone produced in the adjacent physis is replaced by more structurally sound bone and thus already has a high osteogenic potential.

1.3.2   Diaphysis

This area is relatively dormant with respect to osteogenesis in comparison. The bone is relatively avascular and as a result has less remodelling potential, taking a longer time to heal and remodel.

1.3.2.1   Angulation

- In the skeletally immature, 75% of the angular remodelling occurs in the physis.

- The concave side grows more rapidly to align the physis so as to become perpendicular to the long axis of the shaft.
- Within the diaphysis, around 20% of the remodelling of angulation occurs with increasing pressure i.e. compression, on the concave side, stimulating growth (Wolff's law).

1.3.2.2 Length

- Overgrowth has been recognised in both femoral and tibial fractures. Femoral overgrowth is independent of age, fracture level or position.
- Tibial overgrowth is age dependent, with the 3–5 year age group most affected.
- The mechanism for this is felt to be an increase in blood flow to the adjacent growth areas in response to the fracture healing process.

1.3.2.3 Rotation

- Remodelling of rotation does not occur to any significant level.

1.4   Types of Fracture in Children

The biomechanics of paediatric bone mean differing patterns of injury are seen from adult bone. Paediatric bone has a lower modulus of elasticity, greater ultimate stress values and is less brittle. This means bone will undergo more 'plastic deformation' before it ultimately fails/fractures. When a bending force is applied to an adult bone, it typically fails on the side under tension, causing a transverse or short oblique type fracture. Given the aforementioned biomechanical properties, paediatric bone may instead fail on the compressive side, manifesting as:

- Buckle or Torus fractures – the tension side remains intact. These are inherently stable fractures and can be treated out of plaster.

- Greenstick fractures – the tension side is disrupted and therefore these fractures may be more unstable.

1.5   Fractures Involving the Physis

Fractures in the metaphyseal/epiphyseal region of bones may also involve the physis. The manner in which the physis is involved is most commonly classified by the Salter-Harris system:

- Salter-Harris I – *physeal separation.*
  - These are fractures through the hypertrophic zone of the physis. They may be difficult to diagnose if undisplaced and only become apparent on follow-up X-rays. They generally have a good prognosis.

- Salter-Harris II – *fracture through the physis, exiting in the metaphysis.*
  - These are the most common fractures.
  - The fragments exit in the metaphysis thus avoiding the germinal zones.
  - The metaphyseal (Thurston Holland) fragment still has periosteum attached to it, aiding reduction.

- Salter-Harris III – *fracture through the physis, exiting in the epiphysis.*
  - By exiting through the epiphysis, these fractures therefore also cause damage to the articular surface. These are typically managed operatively in order to restore both the physis and the articular surface anatomy.

- Salter-Harris IV – *fracture through the physis, epiphysis and metaphysis.*
  - These injuries occur following higher energy impacts. A Thurston Holland fragment is also visible.
  - Given the fracture propagates through the physis, all its zones are affected.

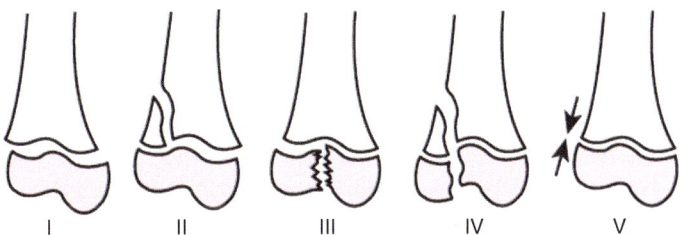

FIGURE 1.1 The Salter-Harris classification (Reprinted with permission from Rockwood and Wilkins' Fractures in Children Lippincott Williams & Wilkins, 2010)

- Salter-Harris V – *crush injury to physis*.
    - These involve a crush injury with no involvement of metaphyseal or epiphyseal components.
    - These are regularly missed on plain radiographs but lead to growth disturbances.
- Salter-Harris (modification by Rang) VI - injury to perichondrial ring of Le Croix usually by direct force such as a lawn mower injury.

SH I and SH II fractures should typically involve the hypertrophic and enchondral ossification zones of the physis and therefore have a low risk of growth disturbance. SH III and SH IV fractures affect the germinal and proliferative zones, therefore inferring a greater risk of growth disturbance (Fig. 1.1).

1.6   Physeal Injuries and Arrest

1.6.1   Epidemiology

- Physeal injuries are common, representing 20–30% of childhood injuries, with the largest proportion of these being in the phalanges.
- The incidence of growth arrest is approximately 1%.

1.6.2   Mechanism

- The physis has only a limited ability to repair, depending on the level of cellular injury within the physis. Partial growth arrest can result from injuries that affect part of the physis but leave the uninjured physis to grow normally. The potential consequences of physeal growth disturbance include the development of angular deformity, limb length inequality and epiphyseal distortion.
- The mechanisms include disruption to the physeal architecture or the formation of bony bridges or physeal bars. This occurs whenever a bridge of bone develops across a portion of physis, tethering the metaphysis and epiphysis. Physeal bars usually require preventative or corrective treatment to minimise long term sequelae.

  Causes of growth disturbance, other than trauma include:

- Infection.
- Blount's disease.
- Irradiation.
- Enchondroma.

1.6.3   Anatomy of the Physis

The physis is arranged in columns of cells or layers. The different layers are:

- *The reserve zone* – this is the layer immediately adjacent to the epiphysis. Cells typically store lipids, glycogen and proteoglycan aggregates for later growth and matrix production. Due to the relatively low cellular activity the oxygen tension is typically low.
- *The proliferative zone* – this has the highest rate of metabolic activity. It is the zone in which chondrocyte proliferation and stacking takes place, and accompanying the high level of metabolic activity an increased oxygen tension.

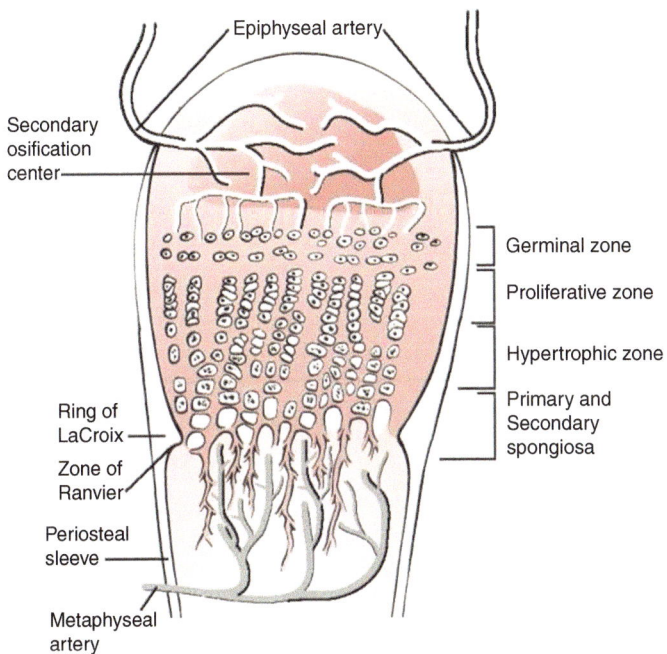

FIGURE 1.2 Diagrammatic representation of a normal physis (With permission form Rockwood and Wilkins' Fractures in Children Lippincott Williams & Wilkins, 2010)

- *The hypertrophic zone* – this zone is itself split into maturation, degeneration and provisional calcification zones.

  - *Maturation zone*: preparation of matrix for calcification and chondrocyte growth.
  - *Degenerative zone*: further preparation of matrix for calcification, and upt ot 5 times chondrocyte growth.
  - *Provisional calcification zone*: chondrocyte death allows calcium release allowing subsequent calcification of the matrix.

- As this area has enlarged cells and lacks significant calcified tissue and collagen, it is more suseptable to traumatic injury (Fig. 1.2).

1.6.3.1 Metaphysis

- Primary spongiosa: osteoblasts align on cartilage bars produced by physeal expansion. This is subsequently mineralised to form woven bone and then remodels to become secondary spongiosa.

- Secondary spongiosa, Internal remodelling to lamellar bone takes place.

- Groove of Ranvier: formed during the first year of life this is a fibrous circumferential ring bridging the epiphysis to the diaphysis. Bring with is mechanical strengthand by supplying chondrocytes to the periphery is responsible for appositional bone growth, and is further supported by the perichondrial fibrous ring of La Croix.

1.6.4   Physeal Growth Arrest

Physeal growth arrest can be classified based on the anatomic relationship to the healthy physis (Figs. 1.3 and 1.4). Bright described this concept in 1974.

- Central.
  - Central arrests are most likely to cause tenting of the articular surface, angular deformity (if eccentrically located) and limb length discrepancy.
- Peripheral.
  - Peripheral arrests primarily cause progressive angular deformity and variable shortening.
- Linear.
  - Linear arrests are through and through, combining the characteristics of both central and peripheral arrests. These injuries most commonly develop after Salter Harris III or IV fractures of the medial malleolus.

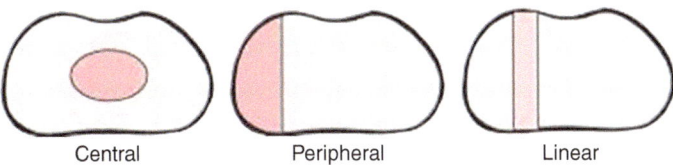

| Central | Peripheral | Linear |

FIGURE 1.3 Example of types of physeal arrest. From *left* to *right* – central, peripheral and linear arrests (Reprinted with permission from Beaty et al (2009) *Rockwood and Wilkins' Fractures in Children*, 7th ed, LWW)

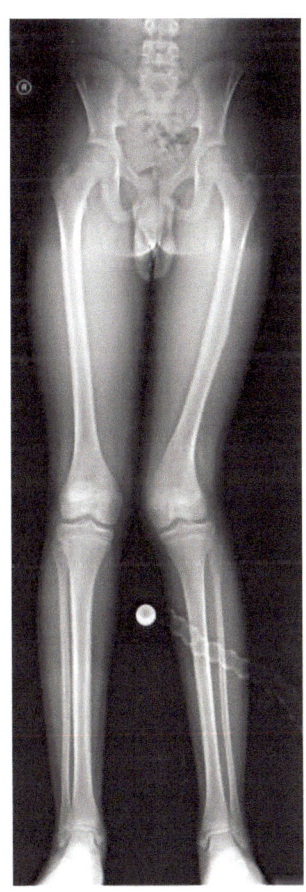

FIGURE 1.4 Long leg standing radiographs showing a left distal femur lateral physeal growth arrest with resultant valgus angulation

1.6.5   Diagnosis

Plain radiographs are often enough to diagnose growth arrest but CT and MRI scans may be needed. Radiological features includes:

- Loss of normal physeal contour.
- Tenting of the articular surface.
- Thinner or thicker physeal area with an indistinct metaphyseal border.
- Asymmetric growth arrest line.

1.6.6   Treatment

1.6.6.1 Partial Physeal Arrest Resection

This involves removal of the bony bridge between the metaphysis and the physis, filling the defect with a material that prevents bone reformation. Considerations before proceeding that should be taken include:

- Type of arrest: central and linear demonstrating the best outcomes.
- Extent of the arrest: if more than 50% of the physeal area is affected, then the physis is unlikely to recover.

Once the anatomy of the physeal bridge has been adequately delineated, the approach can be planned with central lesions being approached through a metaphyseal window. With all resections, the arrest must be carefully removed with minimal damage to the surrounding physis.

The void should then be filled with a material, such as PMMA bone cement, to prevent the bony bridge reforming. Other commonly used materials include:

- Autogenous fat.
- Cranioplast.
- Artificial dura substitute.

1.6.6.2 Repeated Osteotomies

This technique deals with the complication of angular deformity rather than treating the bony bridge. It is not suitable for limb length discrepancies.

1.6.6.3 Completion of Arrest Followed by Correction of Angular Deformity

An alternative is to complete the epiphysiodesis before an angular deformity occurs and then to manage the limb length discrepancy appropriately, either with a limb lengthening procedure or a growth arrest on the contralateral side.

1.6.7   Complications

The major complications of physeal arrest are angular deformity and limb length discrepancy.

Chapter 2
Paediatric Upper Limb Fractures – Shoulder to Elbow

Alex Mulligan and Matthew Barry

2.1 Fractures Around the Shoulder and Humerus

2.1.1 Clavicle Fractures

2.1.1.1 Epidemiology

Clavicle fractures in children are common and represent 8–15% of all paediatric fractures and 90% of obstetric fractures. This is due to its subcutaneous position and the transfer of any force applied to the upper limb passing through this supporting strut. The majority are diaphyseal and can occur through indirect or direct forces e.g. during a fall onto an outstretched hand or direct impact.

A. Mulligan, MBBS, MRCS, MA (Cantab) (✉)
T&O SpR Percivall Pott Rotation, London, UK
e-mail: alex@mulligans.org.uk

M. Barry, MS, FRCS (Orth)
Consultant Orthopaedic and Trauma Surgeon,
Paediatric and Young Adult Orthopaedic Unit,
The Royal London and Barts and The London Children's Hospitals,
Barts Health NHS Trust, London, UK

N.A. Aresti et al. (eds.), *Paediatric Orthopaedic Trauma in Clinical Practice*, In Clinical Practice,
DOI 10.1007/978-1-4471-6756-3_2,
© Springer-Verlag London Ltd. 2015

2.1.1.2 Diagnosis

The child will present with pain and swelling over the fracture site. A full neurological review should be carried out to identify associated brachial plexus injuries. Anteroposterior and oblique cephalic tilt X-rays are usually sufficient to characterise the bony injury. CT should be carried out for medial injuries to assess displacement and determine if the injury is through the growth plate or associated with a sternoclavicular dislocation.

> Special note should be made of vascular compromise, swallowing and airway maintenance in medial injuries due to potential compression of underlying structures

2.1.1.3 Fracture Classification

Allman, in 1967, classified clavicle fractures into three groups based upon anatomical location. Groups I and III were further subdivided by Craig and Neer but the initial anatomical classification is sufficient for describing paediatric fractures.

- Group I – middle third (most common) (Fig. 2.1).
- Group II – lateral third (distal to coracoclavicular ligaments).
- Group III – proximal (medial) third.

2.1.1.4 Treatment and Indications for Surgery

The majority of clavicle fractures can be treated conservatively in a sling for 2–4 weeks, depending on the child's age, followed by mobilization.

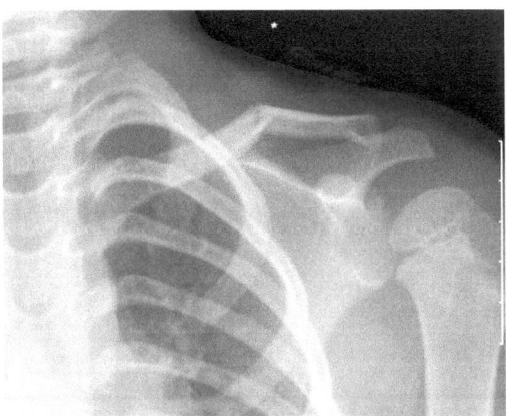

Figure 2.1 Plain radiograph of clavicle fracture, showing a middle third fracture

Indications for surgery include:

- Open fractures.
- Tenting of overlying skin which threatens soft tissue envelope.
- Plexus or vessel impingement, clinically or on imaging.

Open surgery aims to reduce the fracture fragments back into their periosteal sleeve with repair of the ruptured periosteum. This will usually result in a stable reduction and fixation is rarely required.

Medial sternoclavicular joint dislocation or a displaced Salter Harris (SH) I or II fracture should be assessed on CT and undergo closed reduction under general anaesthetic. Unstable reductions can be augmented by open capsular repair.

2.1.1.5 Follow-Up

Fracture clinic review can be carried out at 1 week and 4 weeks post-injury with clinical assessment and mobilization as the shoulder becomes more comfortable. Repeat X-rays are often not required.

Some institutions still use figure of eight bandages to encourage return to full length and alignment as the fracture callus matures. If this is the case, then the child should be reviewed weekly to ensure that no compression complications are developing as result of the bandage position.

2.1.1.6 Complications

- Neurovascular compromise.
- Mal-union.
- Non-union (this is rare and has never been documented in a child under the age of 12 years).
- Pulmonary injury.

2.1.1.7 Synopsis

- Common childhood fractures with a long tradition of successful conservative treatment with sling immobilization.
- Care should be taken with medial injuries as there is a recognized risk of compression of associated structures and therefore more often require reduction in theatre.

2.1.2 Acromio-Clavicular & Sterno-Clavicular Dislocations

Acromio-clavicular (AC) joint disruptions are rare, and when present occur in children over the age of 13. It is important to differentiate between a true AC joint disruption and a fracture. The distal clavicle physis does not ossify till adolescence and so SH I type injuries may be commonly mistaken for AC joint disruptions. They are treated much the same as adults.

Sterno-clavicular (SC) joint disruption is rarer than AC disruptions and similar diagnostic difficulties arise as the

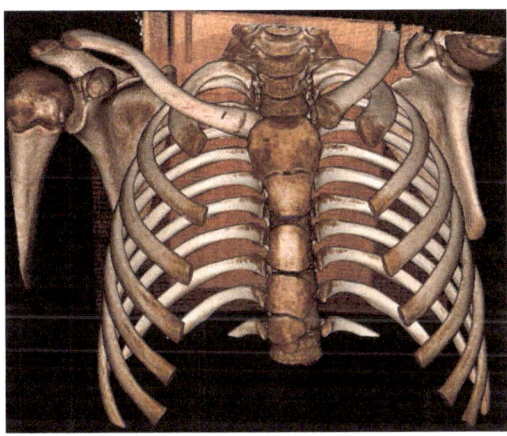

FIGURE 2.2 CT reconstructions in 3D showing a sternoclavicular dislocation

ossification centre at the medial end does not appear until about 16, fusing at around 25 (Fig. 2.2).

2.1.3   Proximal Humerus Fractures

2.1.3.1 Epidemiology

These relatively uncommon injuries occur with an incidence of 1–2 in 1000 and account for approximately 5% of paediatric fractures. They occur most commonly in the adolescent involved in sporting activity through a direct or indirect blow and can involve the after metaphysis (Fig. 2.3), physis or both. The metaphysis is the most commonly affected area in 5–12 year olds due to the rapid growth in this area and the structural weakness in this growing bone. Birth injuries of the proximal humerus are physeal fractures and are often misdiagnosed as glenohumeral dislocations. Ultrasound is useful to confirm a located glenohumeral joint and no fracture treatment is required beyond bandage for analgesia.

2.1.3.2 Diagnosis

The older child will present with a consistent traumatic history and the arm held in internal rotation to offload the
deforming force of pectoralis major on the distal fragment.
Range of movement will be limited by pain. Associated injuries including glenohumeral dislocation and neurological
injury should be sought. They can be ruled out with a full set
of anteroposterior, lateral or Y view and axial X-ray views
and detailed neurological examination.

2.1.3.3 Fracture Classification

Proximal epiphyseal humeral fractures were classified by
Neer and Horowiz in 1965 and describe the extent of fracture
displacement:

- Grade I – up to 5 mm displacement.
- Grade II – up to one third displacement.
- Grade III – up to two thirds displacement.
- Grade IV – greater than two thirds displacement.

2.1.3.4 Treatment and Indications for Surgery

Eighty percent of humeral growth occurs at the proximal
humerus. This results in massive potential for remodeling.
Combined with a large range of movement at the glenohumeral joint, good outcomes can be expected for what may
appear to be significant displacement or angulation.

Acceptable displacement:

- Age 1 to 4 – 70° of angulation and any amount of
  displacement.
- Age 5 to 12 – 40–45° of angulation and up to 50% of
  metaphyseal width translation.
- Age >12 – 15–20° of angulation and translation of up to
  one third of metaphyseal width.

FIGURE 2.3 Proximal humerus fracture

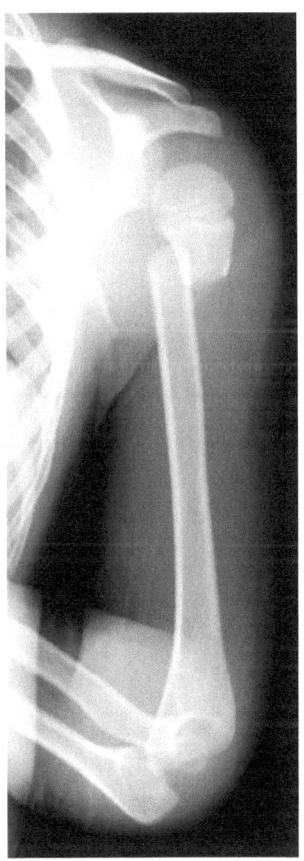

Closed reduction under anaesthetic in theatre is indicated for displacements beyond these ranges.

Indications for surgery include:

- Open fractures.
- Associated neurovascular compromise.
- Salter Harris III or IV fractures with displacement.
- Irreducible fracture dislocations.
- Displaced lesser tuberosity fractures.

Fixation in unstable fractures is maintained with percutaneous smooth Kirschner wires for epiphyseal and high metaphyseal fractures and intramedullary rods for more distal fractures.

2.1.3.5 Follow-Up

In patients up to the age of 5 years, a sling can be used for 5–7 days followed by review in fracture clinic and mobilization. In the over 5 s, the sling can be maintained for 2–3 weeks followed by fracture clinic review and mobilization.

Reduced range of movement associated with stiffness or deformity in the paediatric patient will resolve with time and remodelling in the vast majority of cases. If there is functional deficiency at the 4–6 week review, then further review at 3–6 months for repeat examination will often reveal resolution of their symptoms.

2.1.3.6 Complications

- Proximal humeral varus.
- Limb length inequality.
- Loss of motion.
- Inferior glenohumeral subluxation.
- Osteonecrosis.
- Nerve injury.
- Growth arrest.

2.1.3.7 Synopsis

- Neer Grade I and II injuries almost invariably do well with conservative measures due to their remodeling potential.
- Grade III and IV injuries may have some residual angulation or shortening but even these are well tolerated.

2.2   Fractures Around the Elbow

2.2.1   Supracondylar Fractures

2.2.1.1 Epidemiology

Supracondylar fractures account for 60% of all elbow fractures and 30% of all paediatric extremity fractures. The peak age of occurrence is 5–7 years with a male to female ratio of 3:2. Nerve injury occurs in 7% and vascular injury in 1%. Ninety percent are extension type fracture pattern.

2.2.1.2 Diagnosis

History – Fall onto an outstretched hand or from a height is typical. Depending on the mechanism of injury, consider other associated injuries (wrist fracture) and the possibility of non-accidental injury (NAI) should be considered in the younger child.
Examination – *Look* for swelling, bruising, deformity and any associated wounds. *Feel* for tenderness, pulses, capillary refill and assess neurological status.

- Anterior interosseus nerve – most commonly injured nerve.

  – absent 'OK' sign.

- Median nerve.

  – Motor: thenar muscle.
  – Sensory loss: palmar surface index finger.

- Radial nerve.

  – Motor: wrist drop.
  – Sensory loss: first dorsal web space.

- Ulnar nerve.

  – Motor: interossei.
  – Sensory: palmar surface little finger.
  – May be an iatrogenic injury.

Move fingers through passive flexion and extension to assess the compartment pressures of the forearm. Movement of the elbow is difficult owing to pain, and this pain is significantly worsened in the presence of compartment syndrome. The joints above and below should be examined to exclude associated injuries.

The cold, non-perfused and pulseless (on palpation or Doppler) forearm in the context of a supracondylar fracture should be treated as a vascular emergency

---

2.2.1.3 Fracture Classification

Supracondylar fractures were classified by Gartland in the 1950s, and further modified by Wilkins to include rotational deformity.

- Type I – undisplaced.
- Type II – displaced but some cortical contact.
  - IIA – no rotational deformity.
  - IIB – rotational deformity present.
- Type III – displaced with no cortical contact (Fig. 2.4).

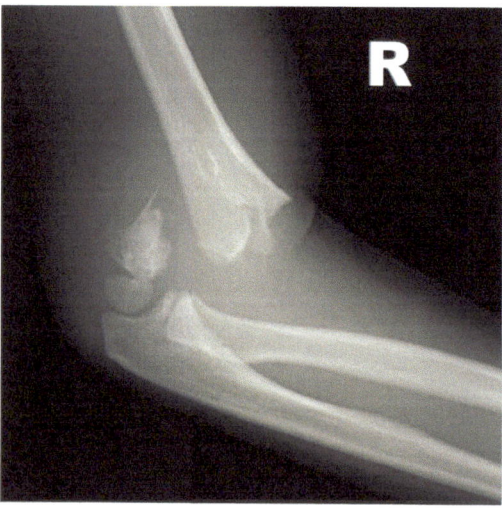

Figure 2.4 Gartland 3 supracondylar fracture

2.2.1.4 Treatment and Indications for Surgery

Initial management includes analgesia, splintage in a back-slab at 20–40°, elevation and regular re-assessment.
Treatment by classification:

- Type I: collar and cuff or above elbow cast in 90° of flexion with neutral forearm for 2–3 weeks.
- Type II: conservative vs surgical depending on age and extent of displacement. Surgical intervention with manipulation under anaesthetic and percutaneous K-wire fixation.
- Type III: attempt at closed reduction under anaesthetic and K-wire fixation. Progress to open reduction and K-wiring if unable to reduce or deteriorating distal vascularity on reduction.

2.2.1.5 Controversies:

Vascular deficit

The white and pulseless limb should be treated as a vascular emergency with emergent reduction and stabilization in theatre followed by reassessment of vascularity. Ongoing signs of ischaemia should prompt opening and vascular exploration and intervention as required.
The pink, pulseless limb remains more controversial.

- There remains the recognized potential for progression to white and pulseless, so the vascular surgeons should be informed early.
- The child should undergo urgent but non-emergent reduction and fixation followed by observation for at least 48 h.
- Loss of Doppler signal or clinical deterioration intra- or post-operatively should prompt vascular exploration.
- Absent pulses at discharge with a perfused hand has been shown to have no adverse effect on long-term functional outcome.

Number and orientation of wires

- Crossed wires have been traditionally held to be more stable but the medial wire can result in direct or indirect injury of the ulnar nerve.
- With good technique lateral-entry wires have been shown to be just as stable under physiological loads as long as the wires:
    - Are at least 2 mm in diameter.
    - Diverge to engage both medial and lateral columns.
    - The inferior wire engages the cortices at the olecranon fossa.
    - The construct is tested for stability in rotation on the table.

With both techniques, iatrogenic ulnar nerve injury remains rare.

2.2.1.6 Follow-Up

In general, K wires can be removed at 4 weeks and if necessary, the cast can be retained for a further 2 weeks. Final fracture clinic review is at 10–12 weeks to assess range of movement and assess carrying angle.

2.2.1.7 Complications

Early:

- Compartment syndrome.
- Neurological injury.
- Vascular injury.
- Pin site infections.

Late:

- Stiffness.
- Malunion/cubitus varus (gunstock deformity).

2.2.1.8 Synopsis

- Common paediatric trauma injury.
- Vascular compromise associated with forearm compartment syndrome and should prompt urgent or emergent reduction and fixation with reassessment of vasculature.
- Gartland Type I fractures most commonly treated non-surgically, Type II and III commonly require manipulation under anaesthetic and K wire fixation.
- Medial and lateral wires or multiple lateral-entry wires are both effective.

2.2.2   *Condylar Fractures*

2.2.2.1 Epidemiology

Lateral condyle fractures are more common than medial fractures, and condylar fractures are the second most common elbow fracture in children which requires operative intervention. There is a similar age and sex distribution as supracondylar fractures. Condylar fractures can heal slowly, may displace late and have a tendency to non-union. For this reason there must be a high index of suspicion and low threshold for intervention in these injuries.

2.2.2.2 Diagnosis

History and examination will identify a painful elbow often in the context of a fall from height. Appropriate initial X-rays include anteroposterior and lateral views. In the presence of an elevated fat pad and a consistent history but with no obvious displaced fracture on the initial views, an oblique view X-ray may be helpful.

2.2.2.3 Fracture Classification

Lateral condyle fractures were classified by Milch in 1955 (Figs. 2.5 and 2.6).

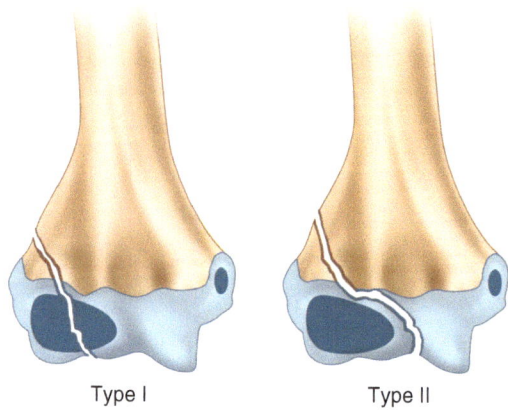

Type I   Type II

FIGURE 2.5 Diagram of lateral condyle fractures

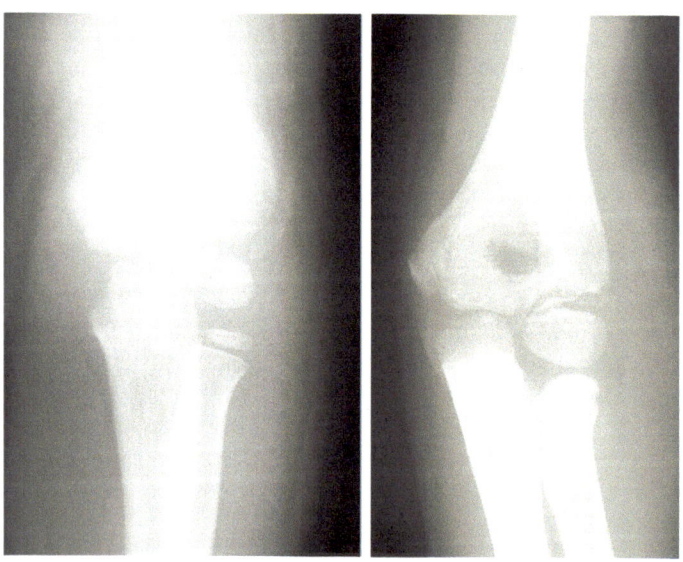

FIGURE 2.6 Plain radiographs of lateral condyle fractures. The
image on the left shows a Milch 1 fracture and on the right a Milch
2 fracture

- Type I – fracture involves the ossification centre of the capitellum and will enter the joint lateral to the trochlear ridge.
- Type II – fracture extends into the non-ossified trochlear, through or medial to trochlear ridge.

Jakob and Kilfoyle further classified lateral and medial condylar injuries respectively according to the extent of displacement:

- Stage I – non-displaced (<2 mm), articular surface intact.
- Stage II – 2–4 mm displacement, articular surface disrupted.
- Stage III – displaced and rotated.

2.2.2.4 Treatment and Indications for Surgery

Treatment by Jakob/Kilfoyle Classification:

Stage I:

- Posterior splint with lateral gutter in 90° flexion and neutral rotation.
- Fracture clinic weekly, with AP, lateral and oblique XOA.
- Mobilise at 4–6 weeks if clinically and radiologically united.

Stage II and III:

- Open reduction and internal fixation (Fig. 2.7).
- Consider intraoperative arthrography.
- Fracture clinic in 1 week, XOA + reinforce cast.
- Fracture clinic in 4–6 weeks for XOA + wires out + mobilise.
- If any concern regarding osteonecrosis or growth disturbance then follow-up for up to 3 years.

2.2.2.5 Complications

Early:

- Compartment syndrome.
- Neurological injury.
- Vascular injury.
- Pin site infections.

FIGURE 2.7 K-wire fixation
of a lateral condyle fracture

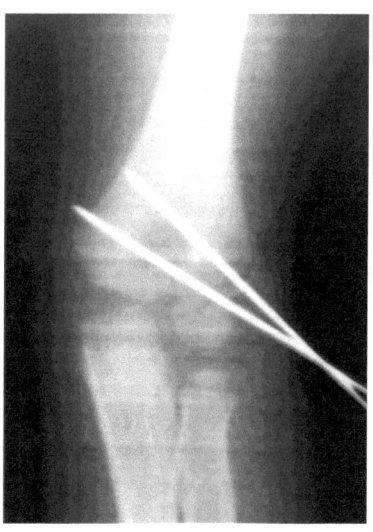

Late:

- Malunion.
- Osteonecrosis – incidence reduced by maintaining posterolateral soft tissue attachments during open approaches, as the blood supply to the lateral condyle mainly originates posteriorly.
- Stiffness.

2.2.2.6 Synopsis

- Second most common operative paediatric elbow fracture.
- High index of suspicion in context of consistent history and examination and low tolerance for obtaining oblique X-ray views.
- Heal slowly, displace late and tendency for non-union.

2.2.3 Apophyseal Injuries

2.2.3.1 Epidemiology

Medial epicondyle fractures account for 10% of all paediatric elbow fractures. The typical age at presentation is between 9 and 14 years old. They are more common in boys with a M:F ratio of 4:1. Up to 50% will present with an associated elbow dislocation and the vast majority are thought to happen alongside a dislocation. 15–20% are incarcerated in the joint.

2.2.3.2 Diagnosis

The child will present with a history of trauma with or without dislocation, or in the case of throwing athletes a popping sensation followed by immediate pain. They are caused by a valgus stress and avulsion of the medial epicondyle by the flexor-pronator muscle mass. X-rays may show widening of the apophysis, displacement of the epicondyle or incarceration of the epicondyle within the joint.

2.2.3.3 Fracture Classification

Beaty and Kasser/Rang Classification:

- Type I – undisplaced or minimally displaced.
- Type II – displaced greater than 5 mm.
- Type III – incarcerated in joint (without dislocation on X-ray).
- Type IV – incarcerated in joint with elbow dislocation on X-ray.

2.2.3.4 Treatment and Follow-Up

Most epicondyle fractures can be managed non-operatively with a sling for comfort and early mobilization.
    Absolute indications for surgery:

- Incarceration of epicondyle within the joint.

    Relative indications for surgery:

- Associated ulnar nerve palsy.
- High level sports-person or expected high demand.
- Joint instability.
- Significant displacement – more than 10 mm.

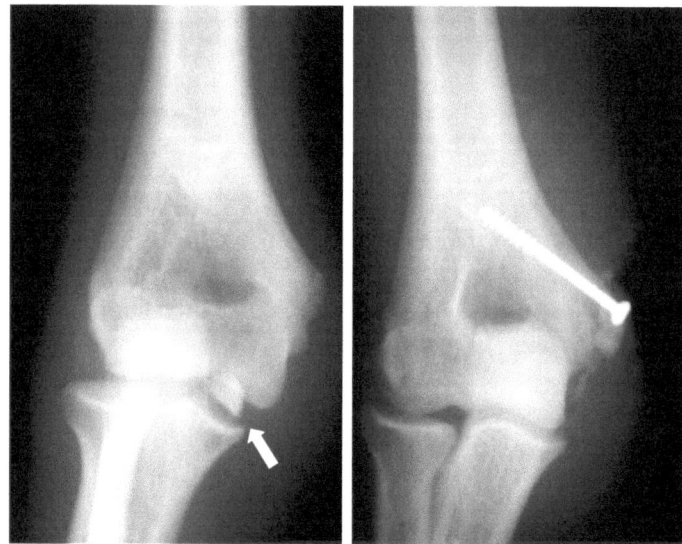

FIGURE 2.8 Operative fixation of apophyseal injury. The arrow on the left hand picture points towards the incarcerated epicondyle

On the medial side, the location of the ulna nerve should be ascertained to confirm it is not trapped in the fracture site. In younger children, two divergent K-wires can be used to hold the fragment reduced. The arm should go into a long cast splint for 3–5 weeks followed by wire removal and mobilization. In older children, a single screw could be used and mobilization started as soon as the soft tissues have started to settle (Fig. 2.8).

2.2.3.5 Complications

Early

- Compartment syndrome.
- Neurological injury.
- Vascular injury.
- Pin site infections.

Late:

- Malunion.
- Stiffness.

> Medial epicondyle fractures are almost always in the context of elbow dislocations. Stiffness following operative or non-operative management should often be regarded as a feature of the capsular disruption during dislocation and patients and families should be counselled regarding this at the first opportunity

2.2.4   Transphyseal Fractures

2.2.4.1 Epidemiology

These fractures are rare, are found most commonly in infants under the age of 2 years and can occur as the result of a birth injury. Diagnosis is challenging in this age group due to the predominantly cartilaginous distal humerus. There may be translation of the ulna relative to the humeral shaft. Ultrasound can be helpful to confirm the diagnosis.

2.2.4.2 Fracture Classification

Delee classification:

- Group A – infants up to 12 months – Salter Harris Type I.
- Group B – 12 months to 3 years – Salter Harris Type I-II.
- Group C – 3–7 years – Salter Harris Type II.

2.2.4.3 Treatment and Follow-Up

Identification of this injury type, especially in infants younger than 2 years old, should result in prompt paediatric review as the rates of NAI, either confirmed or suspected, have been as high as 50% in some series. Operative intervention is occasionally needed and is similar to supracondylar fractures with manipulation under anaesthetic and K-wiring.

Key References

Omid R, Choi PD, Skaggs DL. Supracondylar humeral fractures in children. J Bone Joint Surg Am. 2008;90:1121–32.

Weller A, et al. Management of the pediatric pulseless supracondylar humeral fracture: is vascular exploration necessary? J Bone Joint Surg Am. 2013;95(21):1906–12.

Beaty J, et al. Supracondylar fractures of the distal humerus. In: Rockwood and Wilkins fractures in children. Philadelphia: Lippincott Williams & Wilkins; 2006.

Shrader W. Pediatric supracondylar fractures and pediatric physeal elbow fractures. Orthop Clin N Am. 2008;39:163–71.

Chapter 3
Paediatric Upper Limb Fractures – Forearm to Hand

Alex Mulligan and Matthew Barry

3.1 Fractures Around the Forearm

3.1.1 Epidemiology

Fractures of the distal radius account for approximately 23 % of all paediatric fractures with shaft fractures accounting for 5 % of all fractures. Proximal forearm fractures are less common and account for only 1 % of all fractures. Considering both bone forearm fractures, distal third fractures are the most common site and account for 75 % of fractures, mid third fractures occur in about 20 % and proximal third fractures are uncommon and account for only 5 %.

In most cases, forearm fractures in children are sustained as the result of a fall on an outstretched arm. Other mechanisms of injury include a direct blow during sporting activities.

———————

A. Mulligan, MBBS, MRCS, MA (Cantab) (✉)
T&O SpR Percivall Pott Rotation, London, UK
e-mail: alex@mulligans.org.uk

M. Barry, MS, FRCS (Orth)
Consultant Orthopaedic and Trauma Surgeon,
Paediatric Orthopaedic Surgeon, The Royal London
and Barts and The London Children's Hospitals,
Barts Health NHS Trust, London, UK

N.A. Aresti et al. (eds.), *Paediatric Orthopaedic Trauma in Clinical Practice*, In Clinical Practice,
DOI 10.1007/978-1-4471-6756-3_3,
© Springer-Verlag London Ltd. 2015

35

Non-accidental injury should always be considered and if there is any doubt as to the mechanism of injury, early involvement of the paediatric service is mandatory.

3.1.2   Diagnosis

The child presents with a history of trauma and on examination is found to have pain, tenderness, swelling and often deformity at the site of injury. Investigation with an X-ray of both bones and including the wrist and elbow will be required to characterise the nature of the fracture, and to exclude other fractures or associated injuries such as a radial head dislocation. Further investigations are rarely indicated unless the history and examination is suggestive of a pathological fracture or non-accidental injury.

The examination of the limb must include an assessment of the soft tissues – any wound on the forearm must be assumed to be in communication with the fracture site and the management of an open fracture may follow a different path. A careful neurovascular examination is required and although vascular injuries are rare in children's forearm fractures, neurological injuries have been reported to occur in up to 15% of cases, with the median nerve the most commonly injured nerve.

3.1.3   Olecranon Fractures

3.1.3.1 Fracture Classification

Olecranon fractures have been classified to take account of both acute fractures and chronic repetitive injuries to the apophysis as the result of sporting activity, in particular tennis, gymnastics or baseball pitching.

- Type I – apophysitis.
- Type II – stress fracture.
- Type IIIa – apophyseal avulsion.
- Type IIIb – apophyseal-metaphyseal fracture.

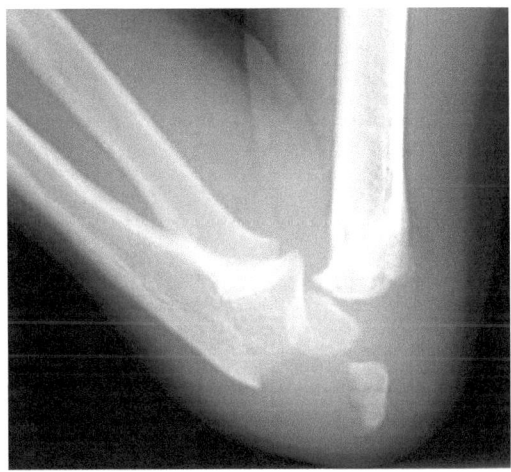

FIGURE 3.1 Plain radiograph of olecranon fracture

Isolated olecranon fractures in children are uncommon. Separation of the olecranon apophysis has been reported but it is rare. Associated injuries such as lateral condyle or radial neck fractures are common and need to be excluded by careful examination of the radiographs (Fig. 3.1).

3.1.3.2 Treatment and Indications for Surgery

The majority (80%) of fractures are undisplaced and can be managed with a plaster cast alone. The elbow should be immobilised for a period of 3–6 weeks, depending on the age of the child.

Indications for surgery:

- Open fracture.
- Fracture displacement with loss of active elbow extension.

Open reduction aims to reduce any articular surface incongruency, and reduction is held with longitudinal Kirschner wires with a supporting figure-of-eight tension band suture as required.

3.1.3.3 Follow-Up

Following operative reduction and fixation, the elbow should be protected in a cast for 4–6 weeks with encouragement of wrist and hand mobilization. Longitudinal K-wires are removed at 8–10 weeks.

3.1.3.4 Complications

- Delayed union.
- Nerve injury.
- Elongation / spur formation resulting in limits to extension.
- Loss of reduction in conservatively managed cases.

3.1.4   Radial Head and Neck Fractures

3.1.4.1 Fracture Classification

Proximal radius fractures in children more commonly affect the neck rather than the head. When the physis is involved it is most commonly a Salter Harris Type II fracture. Neck fractures are classified according to the angular deformity and displacement by Metaizeau:

- Grade 1 – 0° angulation with translation.
- Grade 2 – less than 30° angulation.
- Grade 3 – 30 to 60° angulation.
- Grade 4a – 60 to 80° angulation.
- Grade 4b – greater than 80° angulation (Fig. 3.2).

3.1.4.2 Treatment and Indications for Surgery

Many radial neck fractures are undisplaced and can be managed conservatively. Up to 30° of angulation at the radial neck is acceptable (Grade 1–2). Early mobilisation with a collar and cuff sling for comfort should be encouraged.

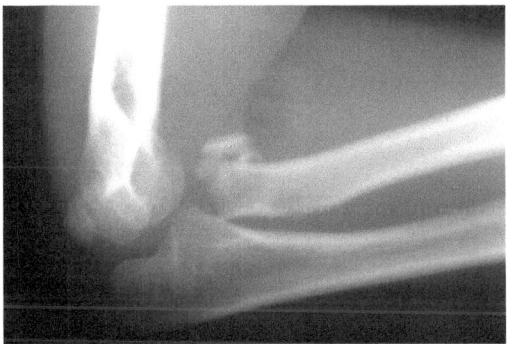

FIGURE 3.2 Plain radiograph of radial neck fracture

The sling can generally be discontinued after a period of 2–3 weeks, as comfort allows. A return to normal function can be anticipated although full elbow extension may take a month or two to recover.

Indications for Surgery:

• More than 30° of angulation at the radial neck (Grade 3–4).

Stable closed reduction can be treated in a collar and cuff in a similar way to minimally displaced fractures. Open reduction should be avoided where possible, using a K-wire to joystick the head fragment back into place or a retrograde elastic nail or Ilizarov wire to flip the fragment back into position.

3.1.4.3 Follow-Up

If percutaneous wires are left in situ, then the elbow will require protection in a cast for 4 weeks before removal of the wire. If a retrograde IM rod has been used, then the mobilization can be initiated immediately and the rod removed at 2–3 months after the initial surgery.

3.1.4.4 Complications

- Decreased range of movement (pronation > supination > extension > flexion).
- Radial head overgrowth.
- Premature physeal closure.
- Radial head osteonecrosis.
- Neurological injury (particularly the posterior interosseous nerve).
- Radioulnar synostosis.
- Myositis ossificans.

3.1.4.5 Synopsis

- Surgical intervention is determined by extent of displacement.
- Up to a quarter of patients will have a poor result regardless of treatment, complaining of reduced range of movement.
- Younger patients with less initial displacement and early, closed treatment, will tend to do better.

3.1.5 Monteggia Type Injuries

3.1.5.1 Fracture Classification

Combined proximal ulnar fracture and radial head dislocation is well recognised in the paediatric population and after any forearm or elbow injury, the position of the radial head in relation to the capitellum must be determined on radiographs.

> An intact radiocapitellar line should be sought on two orthogonal views of the elbow when any ulnar fracture or deformation is identified. Successful treatment is confirmed by radial head reduction demonstrated in the same way on two views.

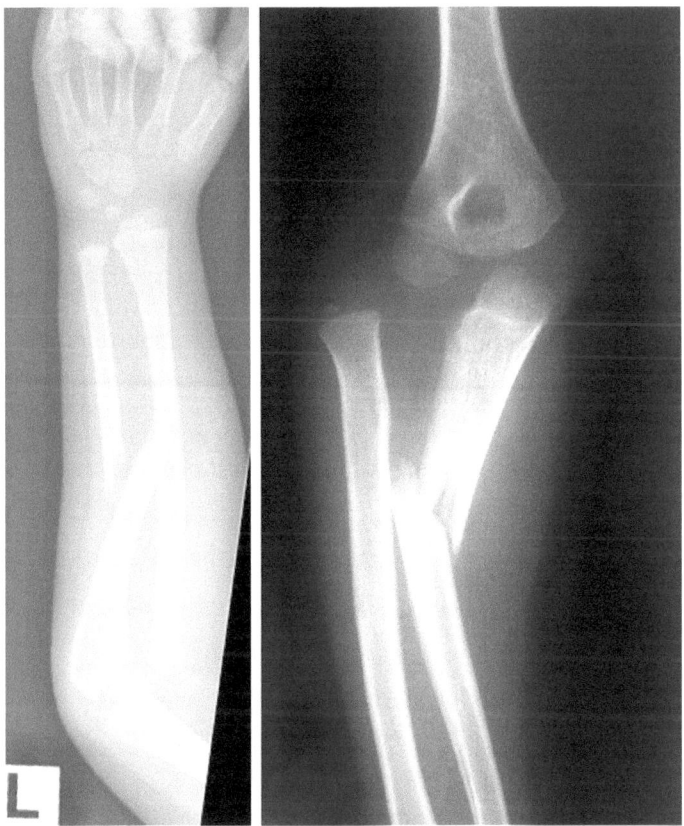

FIGURE 3.3 Bado type I and III Monteggia fracture

The most common classification of the Monteggia lesion is the one proposed by Bado in 1962:

- Type I – anterior dislocation of radial head (70%).
- Type II – posterior dislocation of radial head (6%).
- Type III – lateral dislocation of radial head (23%).
- Type IV – dislocation of the radial head with radial neck fracture (1%) (Fig. 3.3).

3.1.5.2 Treatment and Indications for Surgery

By definition, a Monteggia fracture has an associated radial head dislocation and therefore (after exclusion of a congenital or chronic dislocation) all Monteggia fractures require surgery to re-align the ulna and reduce the dislocation.

Closed reduction of the angulated ulnar fracture will enable stable reduction of the dislocated radial head in almost all acute Monteggia fractures. If the radial head is irreducible, then it will require open exploration to dislodge and repair an obstructing annular ligament.

Radial head instability following successful reduction will be due to recurrent angulation at the ulnar fracture site and requires stabilisation of the fracture with plating, K-wires or intramedullary rods/wires.

3.1.5.3 Follow-Up

The elbow is protected in a cast for 4–6 weeks followed by mobilisation. Wires can be removed in clinic at 4 weeks and plates or rods removed as a day case at 2–3 months.

3.1.5.4 Complications

- Nerve inury (radial nerve 10–20% in Types I and III).
- Myositis ossificans.

3.1.5.5 Synopsis

- Associated radial head dislocation should always be ruled out with an intact radiocapitellar line on AP and lateral films in any ulnar fracture.

3.1.6   Radial and Ulnar Shaft Fractures

3.1.6.1 Fracture Classification

Fractures of the radius and ulna are generally classified by the position of the fracture – proximal, mid or distal third (Fig. 3.4). The use of general fracture classifications such as system proposed by the AO Foundation is an alternative.

3.1.6.2 Treatment and Indications for Surgery

Acceptable deformity:

- Angular deformity – 10° correction per year with degree of acceptable angulation being inversely proportional to distance from the physis.
- Bayonet apposition – up to 1 cm in children <10 years old.
- Rotational deformity and deformity in patients >10 years old should not be accepted.

Closed reduction in a well molded above elbow cast with the forearm in a fracture appropriate orientation provides symptomatic control and allows for a significant improvement in fracture position. The child's age, compliance and injury extent will determine the need for general anaesthesia, sedation or gas and air with analgesia.

Indications for open surgery:

- Unstable/unacceptable fracture reduction after closed reduction.
- Open fracture/compartment syndrome.
- Floating elbow.
- Refracture with displacement.
- Segmental fracture.
- Age (girls >14 years old, boys >15 years old).

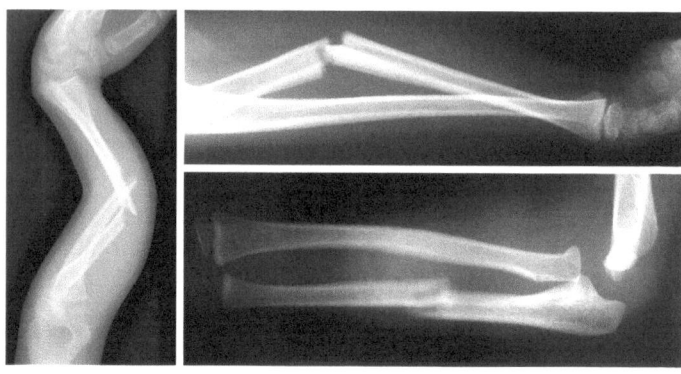

FIGURE 3.4 Plain radiographs of a both bone forearm fracture, an isolated radial fracture and an isolated ulna fracture

Routine operative/open reduction and fixation is with flexible intramedullary nails (elastic nails). These provide effective reduction control while reducing the extent of open dissection, rate of neurovascular injuries, length of surgery and complications associated with future metalwork removal. Indications for plate osteosynthesis include significant comminution or an unstable fracture configuration with potential for shortening.

3.1.6.3 Follow-Up

After a closed reduction or after an open reduction and plate osteosynthesis, an above elbow cast should be maintained for 4–6 weeks. With the cast on, finger movements should be encouraged. At 4 weeks and with radiological signs of union, it may be possible to convert to a short, below elbow cast for the final 2 weeks. After stabilisation, a cast is not strictly required as the fractures are well stabilised but in practice, a short below elbow cast for 2 weeks is used to provide some pain relief. With a short cast, elbow and finger movements should be encouraged. Plates and elastic nails should be removed once the fractures have solidly united and typically this is after 4–6 months. If at the time of the initial operation the end of the elastic nail has not been buried, then it will need to be removed earlier at about 6 weeks and some additional protection may be required.

3.1.6.4 Complications

- Refracture.
- Malunion.
- Synostosis.
- Compartment syndrome.
- Nerve injury.

3.1.7   Distal Radius Fractures

3.1.7.1 Fracture Classification

Fractures of the distal radius are generally classified by their site (metaphyseal or physeal) and whether the fracture is incomplete (e.g. torus, buckle or greenstick) or complete. The complete metaphyseal fracture may be angulated and / or translated at the fracture site. General fracture classifications such as the system proposed by the AO Foundation can also be used.

Physeal fractures of the distal radius are most commonly Salter & Harris Type I or II and about 50% of cases will have an associated fracture of the distal ulna. With a fall onto an outstretched arm, the epiphysis will usually displace dorsally however volar displacement can also occur.

3.1.7.2 Treatment and Indications for Surgery

Incomplete fractures can be treated in a removable splint with early mobilization from 2 to 3 weeks and return to normal activity from 4 weeks. Minimally displaced complete fractures can be immobilized in a below elbow cast for 4–6 weeks depending on the child's age.

> Care must be taken not to label a bicortical fracture (unstable) as a unicortical/buckle/greenstick fracture (stable). The former requires more protection in a complete cast whereas the latter can be treated in a removable splint.

Indications for Surgery:

- Off ended fractures.
- Significant angulation (>20–30°).
- Displaced fracture through physis.

Closed reduction and percutaneous pinning with a smooth 1.6 mm K-wire for unstable reductions is the surgical intervention of choice.

3.1.7.3 Complications

- Malunion.
- Nonunion.
- Cross-union.
- Refracture.
- Growth disturbance.

3.2 Fractures Around the Carpus

3.2.1 Scaphoid Fractures

3.2.1.1 Epidemiology

Scaphoid fractures are the most common paediatric carpal fractures but are still relatively rare accounting for less than half a percent of all upper limb fractures. Distal pole extra-articular fractures are classically held to be the most common. More recent series have suggested that waist fractures are becoming more common, possibly associated with increasing body mass index and participation in higher velocity sports, bringing them more in line with the adult distribution. The peak age is at 15 years and they are more common in boys.

3.2.1.2 Diagnosis

The child will present with a history of trauma and swelling in the region of the scaphoid and anatomical snuffbox tenderness. X-rays should include an anteroposterior, lateral and scaphoid series visualizing the scaphoid in all of its axes (Fig. 3.5). If no fracture is seen but the history and examination are consistent, then further clinical review and X-rays should be carried out at 10–14 days. If a fracture is identified at initial or repeat review, then any evidence of displacement should warrant consideration of further imaging with CT to assess the extent of the displacement. If no fracture is found on repeat review but the child continues to have consistent findings on examination, then an MRI should be organized to confirm the diagnosis.

3.2.1.3 Fracture Classification

Scaphoid fractures in children are described anatomically

- Type A – distal Pole.
- Type B – waist.
- Type C – proximal Pole.

3.2.2 Treatment and Indications for Surgery

Undisplaced fractures can be treated in a cast with thumb spica extension for 6–8 weeks followed by review and repeat X-ray in clinic and mobilization if clinically and radiologically united.

Indications for surgery:

- Displacement >1 mm.
- Angulation >10°.
- Non-union.

Closed reduction and percutaneous pinning or screws have been described in the paediatric population but most will require open reduction of the fracture displacement with internal fixation and bone grafting as required.

3.2.2.1 Follow-Up

Casts remain in situ until fracture union on X-ray. Internal screw fixation may allow early mobilization at two weeks but this is dependent upon the child adhering to limited activity. Any percutaneous wires can be removed in clinic at 4–6 weeks. Stiffness often rapidly improves with simple exercises but hand therapy may be required in some cases, especially where percutaneous wires have been used.

3.2.2.2 Complications

- Delayed union, malunion and non-union.
  - Non-union is much rarer in children than in adults. A delayed presentation or a fracture missed on initial X-rays will still often respond to treatment with cast immobilization and go on to union.
- Osteonecrosis.
- Missed diagnosis.

Fractures in the other carpal bones are extremely rare and when identified are almost all treated with non-surgical cast immobilization for a period determined by the child's age. MRI scanning is useful in suspected cases so that the child and family can be reassured and to avoid over-treating.

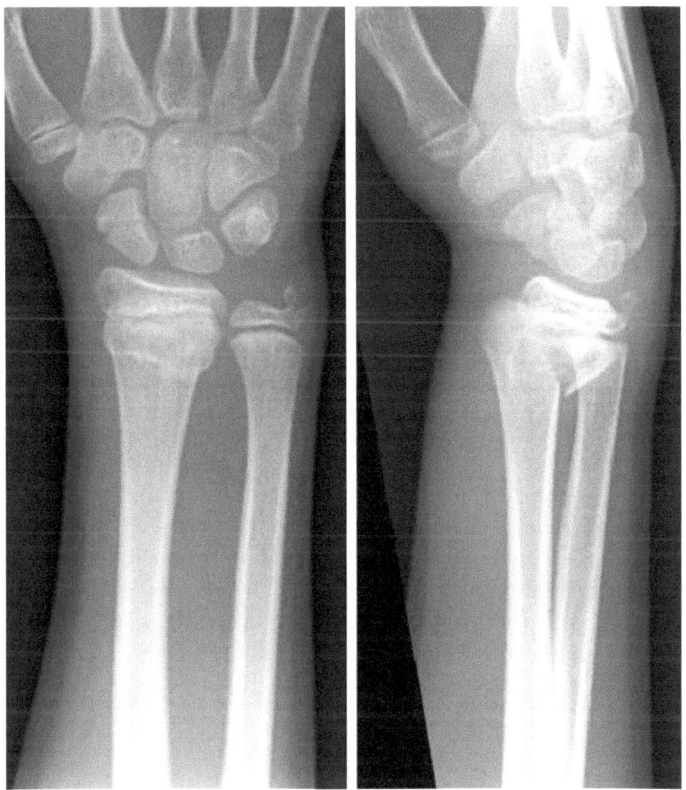

FIGURE 3.5 Plain radiograph of combined distal radius and scaphoid fractures

3.3   Fractures Around the Hand

3.3.1   Epidemiology

Fractures of the hand in children are common, accounting for up to 25% of paediatric fractures. They have a biphasic distribution. Toddlers present following crush injuries with damage to the distal digits whereas adolescents present with proximal phalanx and metacarpal fractures sustained during sport. They are more common in boys and the peak age of presentation in 13 years.

3.3.2   Diagnosis

The child will present with a history of trauma consistent with the area of injury. A younger child may be refusing to play with the affected hand while an older child will be able to localize the area of pain, swelling, tenderness or deformity. Examination should include range of movement and estimation of deformity. In particular it should be noted if there is any scissoring on making a fist, or evidence of rotational deformity. Neurovascular status should be documented (skin wrinkle test in the younger child) and the nail bed inspected for any associated injuries.

X-rays in the anteroposterior, lateral and oblique plains should be carried out. During X-ray review, it is often useful to use the phalangeal line test. A line drawn between the centre of the proximal phalanx head and epiphysis should also pass through the centre of the head of the metacarpal, independent of the flexion at the MCPJ. This line is useful in identifying subtly displaced digit fractures.

3.3.3   Metacarpal Fractures

3.3.3.1 Fracture Classification

The most common metacarpal fracture is the Salter-Harris Type II fracture of the base of the 5th metacarpal.

- Type A – epiphyseal and physeal fractures.
- Type B – neck fractures.
- Type C – shaft fractures.
- Type D – metacarpal base fractures.

3.3.3.2 Treatment and Indications for Surgery

Minimally displaced fractures can be treated in a cast in the safe or Edinburgh position with the MCPJs flexed and the

IPJs extended for 4 weeks followed by mobilization, with or without neighbour strapping for support.

Indications for surgery:

- Any rotational malalignment.
- Angulation at the neck of >15° for index or middle meta-carpals and >30° for ring and little metacarpals.
- Angulation at the shaft of >10°.

Surgical intervention is usually limited to closed reduction under general or local anaesthetic with conscious sedation and splintage. Unstable fractures may require K-wire fixation. Irreducible or significantly displaced epiphyseal or intra-articular fractures may rarely require open reduction and internal fixation.

3.3.3.3 Follow-Up

Immobilisation should be kept in place for 4 weeks and any wires can be removed at 4–6 weeks. Open reduction and stable internal fixation can allow early mobilization at 1 week with a removable splint. Patient guided range of movement exercises can be instituted from 4 weeks with a return to contact activities at 8 weeks.

3.3.3.4 Complications

- Malunion (non-union is rare).
- Osteonecrosis of the metacarpal head.
    - The remodeling potential in this area means that long term joint incongruity is rare.

3.3.4   Thumb Metacarpal Fractures

These most commonly affect the metaphysis or physis.

3.3.4.1 Classification

- Type A – extraphyseal fractures of the metaphysis.
- Type B – Salter-Harris Type II fractures with the metaphy-seal fragment medially.

- Type C – Salter-Harris Type II fractures with the metaphyseal fragment laterally.
- Type D – intraarticular Salter-Harris Type II or IV fractures (equivalent to adult Bennett fractures).

3.3.4.2 Treatment and Indications for Surgery

Up to 30° of angulation can be accepted in extraphyseal fractures and both these and undisplaced physeal fractures can be treated with immobilization in a thumb spica cast for 4–6 weeks.

Indications for surgery:

- More than 30° angulation in extraphyseal fractures.
- Non-anatomical position in Type B, C or D fractures.

Closed or open reduction with percutaneous K-wire fixation is the surgical intervention of choice. A further K-wire can be placed across the 1st and 2nd metacarpals to provide extra neutralizing stability.

3.3.4.3 Follow-Up

With no fixation, cast immobilization should be for 4–6 weeks with repeat X-rays carried out in clinic at weeks 1 and 2 to ensure there is no interval displacement.

Wires can be removed at 4–6 weeks. Young children should be immobilized throughout. Adolescents can start early immobilization from week 1 with a removable splint.

3.3.5   Proximal and Middle Phalanx Fractures

3.3.5.1 Fracture Classification

Classification is based on anatomical position with proximal being the most common (up to 40%)

- Proximal physeal (Salter-Harris Types II (most common), III and IV).

- Shaft.
- Phalangeal neck.
- Intraarticular (condylar).

3.3.5.2 Treatment and Indications for Surgery

Proximal Physcal Fractures

Undisplaced fractures can be treated with immobilization in a safe position with neighbour strapping for 3 weeks followed by mobilization in neighbour strapping for a further 3 weeks.
Indications for surgery:

- Moderate angulation.
- Any rotational or scissoring deformity.
- More than 25% articular involvement or displacement of an epiphyseal fragment by more than 1.5 mm.

Extraphyseal deformity can be treated with closed reduction and splinting. Intraarticular injuries or those around the physis need anatomical reduction by open or closed means and K-wire fixation. A displaced Salter-Harris Type III fragment of the thumb proximal phalanx represents a paediatric Stener-type lesion and often requires open reduction and fixation as it has been pulled through the adductor aponeurosis.

Shaft Fractures

Undisplaced fractures can be treated with immobilization in a safe position with neighbour strapping for 3 weeks followed by mobilization in neightbour strapping for a further 3 weeks.
Indications for surgery:

- More than 30° angulation in a child less than 10 years old.
- More than 20° angulation in a child greater than 10 years old.
- Any rotational deformity.

Surgical intervention is usually limited to closed reduction and percutaneous pinning.

Neck Fractures

Maintenance of reduction in these fractures is difficult due to the pull of local soft tissue structures. Most displaced fractures will require closed reduction and crossed smooth K-wires to maintain the reduction.

Intraarticular/Condylar Fractures

Undisplaced fractures can be treated with immobilization. Anatomical reduction is preferred and any displacement will require closed or open reduction and K-wire fixation. Pilon type fractures with severe articular damage can be treated with dynamic traction.

3.3.5.3 Follow-Up

Cast immobilization after closed reduction without fixation should be reviewed at 1 and 2 weeks post injury with further X-rays in potentially unstable injuries. These include oblique shaft fractures, neck fractures and unicondylar distal fractures.

Immobilisation and any wires are removed at 4 weeks and range of movement exercises encouraged. Periarticular fractures should be reviewed at 4 weeks post mobilization and referred on to hand therapy if recovery is slow.

3.3.6   Distal Phalanx Fractures

3.3.6.1 Fracture Classification

Classification is either physeal or extraphyseal
Physeal:
Dorsal (Mallet Injury)

- Type A – Salter Harris I or II.

- Type B – Salter Harris III or IV.
- Type C – Salter Harris I or II with joint dislocation.
- Type D – Salter Harris fracture with extensor tendon avulsion.

Volar (Reverse Mallet Injury):

- Similar patterns to dorsal injuries but often associated with flexor digitorum longus insertion avulsions with a displaced bony attachment.

Extraphyseal:

- Type A – transverse diaphyseal.
- Type B – longitudinal splitting.
- Type C – comminuted.

3.3.6.2 Treatment and Indications for Surgery

Mildly or moderately displaced fractures can be treated with immobilization in an extension splint for 4–6 weeks
   Indications for surgery:

- Type B dorsal physeal with displacement >50%.
- Type C or D dorsal physeal.

  - Closed or open reduction and internal fixation with K wires.

- Volar type avulsion.

  - These are irreducible fractures that require open reduction and fixation with suture, wires or screws.

- Nailbed open injury or haematoma affecting >50% of the nailbed.

  - These should be decompressed or washed out and repaired with treatment of the underlying fracture as appropriate.

3.3.6.3 Follow-Up

Wires can be removed at 4 weeks and the finger mobilized. Formal hand therapy is rarely required and reserved for those who do not regain function at 3–4 weeks review.

3.3.6.4 Complications

- Imparied nail growth.
- Extensor lag.
- Malunion.
- Nonunion.
- Infection.
- MCPJ extension contracture.

Key References

Cheng J, Ng B, Ying S, Lam P. A 10-year study of the changes in the pattern and treatment of 6,493 fractures. J Pediatr Orthop. 1999;19:344–50.

Younger ASE, Tredwell SJ, Mackenzie WG, Orr JD, King PM, Tennant W. Accurate prediction of outcome after pediatric forearm fracture. J Pediatr Orthop. 1994;14:200–6.

Barry M, Paterson JMH. Flexible intramedullary nails for fractures in children. J Bone Joint Surg. 2004;86-B:947–53.

Williams A, Lochner H. Pediatric hand and wrist injuries. Curr Rev Musculoskelet Med. 2013;6(1):18–25.

Chapter 4
Fractures of the Spine in Children

Edward Britton and Matthew Barry

4.1 Introduction

Paediatric spinal injuries are less common than adult spinal injuries and involve different injury patterns. The evaluation and treatment requires knowledge of the embryology, anatomy, and types of injuries unique to the age of the child. A working knowledge of paediatric spinal ossification centres, as well as the normal findings of the paediatric spinal radiograph, is essential.

Common spinal injuries in the paediatric age group are:

- SCIWORA.
- Atlantooccipital dislocations.
- Epiphysiolysis of the odontoid.
- Cartilage end plate fractures.
- Multiple level fractures.

E. Britton, FRCS (Tr&Orth) (✉)
T&O SpR Royal London Rotation, London, UK
e-mail: emgbritton@gmail.com

M. Barry, MS, FRCS (Orth)
Consultant Orthopaedic and Trauma Surgeon,
Paediatric and Young Adult Orthopaedic Unit,
The Royal London and Barts and The London Children's Hospitals,
Barts Health NHS Trust, London, UK

N.A. Aresti et al. (eds.), *Paediatric Orthopaedic Trauma
in Clinical Practice*, In Clinical Practice,
DOI 10.1007/978-1-4471-6756-3_4,
© Springer-Verlag London Ltd. 2015

- Limbus fractures.
- Lap belt fractures (chance fracture).

This chapter aims to cover the essential knowledge required to identify and treat these injuries appropriately.

4.2   Epidemiology

4.2.1   Incidence

Fractures of the spine in childhood are rare:

- 2–5% of all spine injuries.
- 7 in 100,000 population annually.

It is thought that this may be due to:

1. Increased spinal mobility in children.
2. Increased incidence of missed injuries (several post-mortem studies have suggested that more than 90% of injuries in children may be missed clinically and radiologically because of injuries passing through the physis).

The cause of spinal injuries also differs according to age:

- Children <10 years.

  - Falls (39%).
  - NAI (non-accidental injury).
  - MVA (motor vehicle accident).

- Children >10 years.

  - MVA (52%).
  - Off road vehicles.
  - Falls.
  - Bicycles.

TABLE 4.1

	Child	**Adult**
Multiple level INJ	Less common	Common
Structure injured	Ligaments/soft tissues	Bone
Upper C-spine (%)	70	15
Spinal cord INJ (%)	10	30
SCIWORA (% of SCI)	16	7

4.2.2   Location

Spinal injury patterns in children differ according to age, with injuries in children over the age of 10 years being similar to adults.

This is due to several anatomical factors:

1. Increased ligament laxity resulting in greater flexibility of the spine.
2. Relatively horizontal spine facets in children.
3. Relatively heavy head in relation to the rest of body.
4. Open physes.

These factors affect the site and type of injuries that occur with the majority of spinal injuries in young children occurring in the upper cervical spine (above C3). This is due to the cervical spine fulcrum being more cephalic in children less than 10 years (C2-C3) than in adults (C5-C6). See Table 4.1 for a comparison with adult cervical spine injuries.

Thoracolumbar spinal injuries in children are less common, but within this group they are more common in adolescent children than those younger than 10 years. They also commonly involve multiple levels (16% and often at non adjacent level) due to the elastic intervertebral discs, which distribute forces across multiple levels.

4.3   Anatomy

To be confident in assessing paediatric spines clinically and radiologically, remember the unique ossification patterns of the paediatric spine.

4.3.1   Atlas (C1)

- Three primary ossification centres:

    - Left and right neural arches (ossified at birth).
    - Vertebral body (ossifies at 1 year).

- Fusion:

    - Atlas body and neural arches fuse at 7 years.
    - Spinous processes (neural arch) fuse at 3 years.

4.3.2   Axis (C2)

- Four primary ossification centres at birth (Fig. 4.1):

    - Two odontoid ossification centres fuse in the midline by the 7th foetal month to form one at birth.
    - Vertebral body centre.
    - Two neural arches.

- Secondary ossification centre at the tip of the odontoid appears at 3 years.
- Inferior epiphyseal ring ossifies at puberty.
- Fusion:

    - Spinous processes fuse at 3 years.
    - Axis body and neural arches fuse at 6 years.
    - Axis body and odontoid fuse at 6 years (often visible until age 12).
    - Secondary ossification centre of the odontoid fuses by 25 years, as does the ossification of the inferior epiphyseal ring.

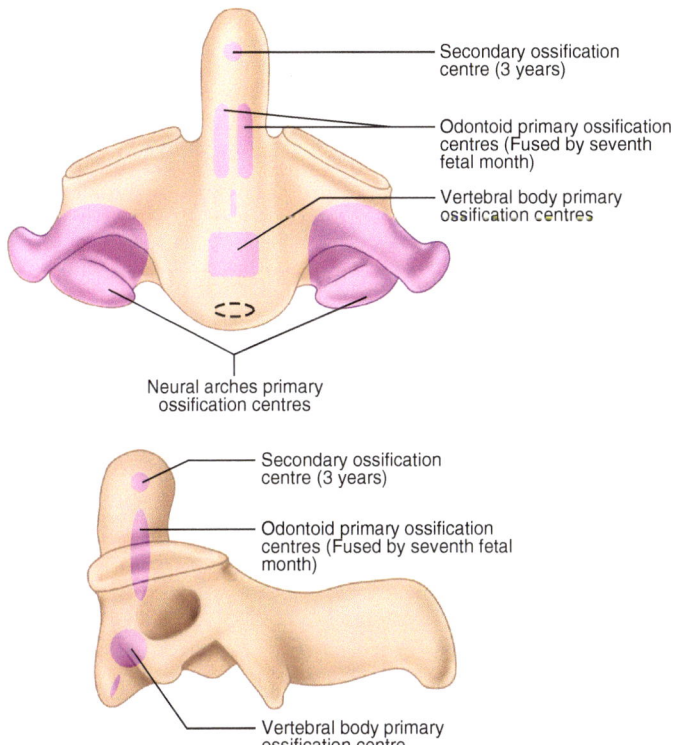

FIGURE 4.1 Ossification centres of odontoid. *1* Secondary ossification centre of odontoid (approximately 3 years), *2* Primary fusion centre of odontoid, *3* Primary ossification centre of vertebral body, *4* Primary ossification centre of of neural arch, *5* Secondary ossification centre of odontoid (approximately 3 years), *6* Primary fusion centre of odontoid, *7* Primary ossification centre of vertebral body

4.3.3 C3-C7

- Five ossification centres at birth:
  - Vertebral body.
  - Two neural arches.
  - Two transverse processes.

- Fusion:

    - Spinous processes fuse by 3 years.
    - Transverse processes fuse to the vertebral body by 6 years.
    - The vertebral body fuses to the neural arches by 6 years.
    - Bifid processes appear at puberty and fuse by age 25.
    - Superior and inferior epiphyseal rings fuse by age 25.

4.3.4   Thoracic and Lumbar Spine

- Adult characteristics and size are present by the age of 10, with similar radiographic examination, except for the open epiphyses.
- Thoracic and lumbar spine ossify and fuse in a similar manner.

4.4   Diagnosis

4.4.1   Imaging

Cervical spine X-rays are not necessary to exclude an injury if the patient:

- Is alert and conversant.
- Has no neurological deficit.
- Has no cervical tenderness.
- Has no painful distracting injury.
- Is not intoxicated.

If the patient does not fall into this bracket, then AP and lateral views are all that are required, as an odontoid view does not aid in making the diagnosis under age 8, and is very difficult to obtain.

Radiographic findings unique to the paediatric cervical spine include:

- Anterior arch of C1 is ossified in only 20% of newborns and may not appear until 1 year of age.
- Atlanto-dens interval is increased in children.
- Retropharyngeal space may be up to 8 mm in children.

- Pseudosubluxation can be a normal finding:
    - C2-C3 is the most common and can be up to 4 mm.
    - C3-C4 is less common and can be up to 3 mm.
    - To distinguish pseudosubluxation from true subluxation, draw Swischuk's line, which should pass no more than 1.5 mm anterior to the interlaminar line of C2 (Fig. 4.2).

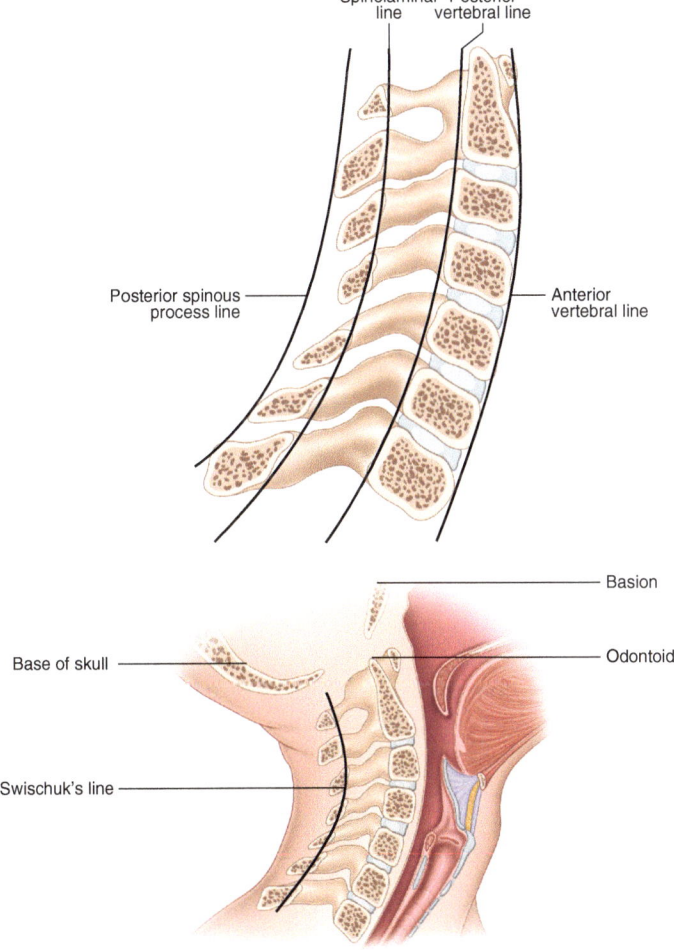

FIGURE 4.2 Radiographic lines of cervical spine. *1* Posterior spinous process line. *2* Spinolaminar line. *3* Posterior vertebral line. *4* Anterior vertebral line

- Cervical lordosis is often absent in children.
- Vertebral bodies are naturally wedged-shaped and can resemble wedge fractures.
- Remember crying can increase soft tissue shadowing markedly (normal is remembered by the mnemonic "2 at 6 and 6 at 2" which referrers to 2 cm soft tissue shadow anterior to C6 and below and 6 mm of shadow in front of C2).

Flexion-extension radiographs add no useful information in the acute setting if the static examination is normal.

4.4.2   Advanced Imaging Studies

MRI directly visualizes the soft tissues and has 87% sensitivity and 100% specificity at predicting instability between the occiput and C1. MRI is therefore very helpful in clearing the cervical spine in the obtunded child, and in this setting can often substitute plain radiographs.

However an MRI scan is poorly tolerated by a conscious child and therefore often requires a general anaesthetic, which carries its own risks.

4.5   Types of Spinal Cord Injury

4.5.1   Spinal Cord Injury Without Radiographic Abnormality (SCIWORA)

This is more common in children than adults, and occurs in 16% of spinal cord injuries in the cervical spine and 7% of spinal cord injuries involving the whole spine in children.

This is thought to be due to the relative increase in flexibility of the immature axial skeleton, compared with the relative resistance to stretching of the spinal cord.

70% of SCIWORAs have complete injuries for which the prognosis is poor.

Typically the injury is apparent on MRI, with spinal cord and surrounding soft tissue oedema at the level of injury.

Immobilisation should be continued until stability has been confirmed.

4.5.2   Atlantooccipital Dislocation

These injuries are often due to hyperextension/distraction injuries and commonly involve the soft tissues and ligaments. They are frequently fatal and most commonly occur following:

- Birth trauma – neck hyperextension in breeched vaginal deliveries resulting in cord transection (stargazing fetus).
- Major blunt trauma.

  Survival is dependent on rapid CPR and ventilatory support.

  Treatment consists of gentle reduction with avoidance of traction and immobilisation with early surgical occiptocervical fusion to allow mobilisation, which would facilitate respiratory support.

4.5.3   Altantoaxial Injuries

These injuries are more common in paediatric patients as opposed to lower cervical spine injuries that are more commonly seen in adult neck injuries.

1. Altantoaxial instability.
   Connective tissue abnormalities such as those in Table 4.2 can cause chronic altanoaxial instability, which will increase the risk of neurological compromise with relatively minor trauma.

   Traumatic altantoaxial instability is secondary to injury to the transverse atlantal ligament. Injury is suspected if the atlanto-dens interval is >5 mm. Treatment is controver-

TABLE 4.2 Diseases associated with atlanto-axial subluxation

Down's syndrome

Larsen syndrome

Reiter syndrome

Juvenile rheumatoid arthritis

Bone dysplasias (e.g. mucopolysaccharidoses, Kneist, multiple epiphyseal dysplasia, achondroplasia, pseudoachondroplasia)

sial with some advocating immediate fusion versus 8–12 weeks of immobilisation.

2. Altas and Axis fractures.
   These are rare and usually heal with appropriate immobilisation.

3. Odontoid fractures.
   These represent 75% of cervical spine fractures in children. Epiphysiolysis of the odontoid (synchondrosis fracture) is the only type of dens fracture occurring under the age of 7. In children these fractures are uncommonly associated with neurological injury due to the relatively large spinal canal at this level (Steel's rule of thirds – 1/3 odontoid process, 1/3 spinal cord, and 1/3 free space).

   Unlike adults, fractures of the odontoid typically heal well and generally require halo vest immobilisation only. An os odontoidenum is thought to represent a non-union of a previous unrecognised odontoid fracture.

4.5.4   Lower Cervical Spine Injuries

After the age of 8, the anatomy of the cervical spine is similar to that of adults and so similar injury patterns are seen. This is due to the joints of Luschka developing by age 8 or 9, which protect against excessive hyperextension.

Injuries in children at this level are generally due to distraction forces and compression burst fractures are rare. Absence of bony pathology is common and separation of cartilage end plates may occur. This may result in spontaneous fusion after immobilisation.

4.5.5   Thoracolumbar Spine Injuries

Spinal injuries at this level in children are generally associated with:

• Vertebral fractures at multiple levels.
• Neurological injuries.
• Other concomitant and serious injuries.

Separation of cartilage end plates are seen in young children, while burst fractures and fracture dislocations occur in adolescents. This change in injury pattern is associated with the incomplete ossification and the horizontal nature of the facet joints seen until age 8.

4.5.6 Limbus Fractures

This is a posterior vertebral epiphyseal injury and can be mistaken for a herniated nucleus pulposus (Fig. 4.3).

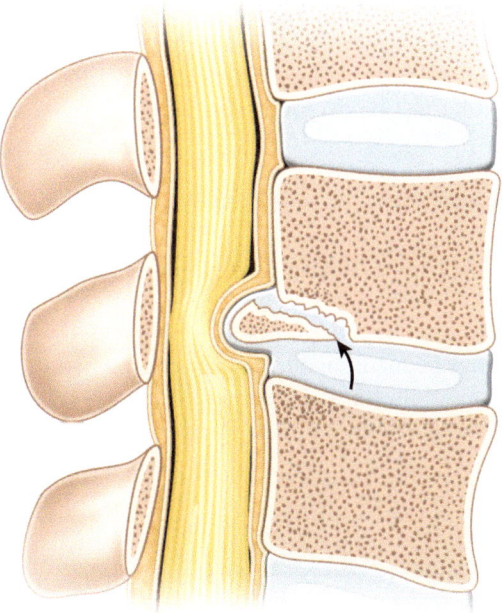

FIGURE 4.3 Diagram demonstrating limbus fracture (*arrow*). Notice the posterior epiphyseal injury that may be mistaken for a herniated disc

4.5.7   Lap-Belt Injury

This injury is the result of a flexion distraction injury of the spine, which results in tension failure of the middle and posterior columns of the spine, and may be purely a ligamentous injury or result in a horizontal *chance fracture*. A resultant paraplegia presents more commonly than in adults and is in up to 30% of cases, and may be explained by the higher centre of gravity in children.

This type of injury is commonly associated with the 'seat belt sign' and abdominal injuries secondary to compression of the aorta, intestinal viscera and abdominal musculature between the seat belt and spinal column. Therefore a high index of suspicion is required for this type of injury, since missed injuries may be life threatening.

Note that CT scans can easily miss these transverse fractures.

Treatment is generally immobilisation and in cases of wide separation of the spine, internal fixation is indicated. Distraction must be avoided (Fig. 4.4).

4.6   Treatment

Treatment of spinal injuries in children is outside the remit of this chapter. Suffice to say that these injuries are serious and should be managed expectantly. A high index of suspicion must always be maintained, and expert opinions sought immediately. Immobilization of the spine will however be discussed as it is often applied on presentation.

4.6.1   Immobilization

Immobilization of a young paediatric spine in a trauma situation must take into account their disproportionately larger heads, so to avoid the risk of kyphosis and anterior translation of the upper cervical spine. This can be achieved by a split mattress, which will recess the occiput.

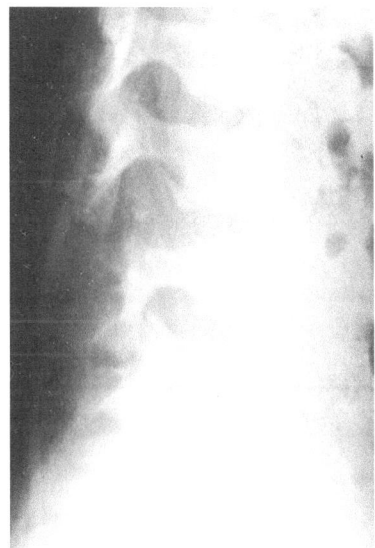

FIGURE 4.4 A 3-year-old male sustained a seat-belt fracture at L1–L2 as a restrained backseat passenger. The lateral view demonstrates spreading and angulation of the spinous process and vertebral bodies, suggesting posterior ligamentous disruption similar to the chance fracture in the adult (figure and legend reprinted with permission from Benson et al. (2009) *Children's Orthopaedics and Fractures*, Springer)

Methods of prolonged immobilization of the paediatric cervical spine are:

- Cervical spine orthoses (Minerva jacket).
- Halo vest.

A cervical spine orthosis only restrict 45% of C1-C2 motion while a halo vest restricts 75%.

Halo vests can be used in patients as young as 2 years. However there are some special considerations:

- Size – often a special order item.
- Location of cranial sutures (4:30 and 7:30).

- Number of pins – usually inversely proportional to the age of the child; up to 10 pins may be necessary in the very young.
- Torque on the pins – the younger the patient, the less torque used (to reduce risk of halo pin penetration).

4.6.2   Complications

Spinal cord injury is less common in younger children (<10) than in older children and in adults; however death from a spinal cord injury occurs more commonly in young children (5.1 times greater under age 11, rather than over 11).

In individuals with spinal trauma, children have a higher incidence (45%) of spinal cord injury than adults. The prognosis however is generally better than in adults, with 74% of partial spinal cord injuries showing significant improvement and 59% achieving a complete recovery, while complete spinal cord injuries behave similarly to adults with little prospect of improvement.

SCIWORA is much more common in children and accounts for approximately 16% of all spinal cord injuries. The explanation for this is also thought to be due the relatively increased flexibility of the spinal column especially in comparison with the spinal cord.

Chapter 5
The Paediatric Hip and Pelvis

Nick A. Aresti and Manoj Ramachandran

5.1 Introduction

Pelvic fractures in children are rare and differ considerably from adult fractures. They are generally either sport related avulsion fractures or fractures related to high-energy trauma. Hip fractures are even less common and are also related to high-energy trauma. They may have significant complications. This chapter aims to separately classify childhood pelvic, acetabular and hip fractures and aid you in their diagnosis and treatment.

N.A. Aresti, MBBS, BSc (Hons), MRCS (✉)
T&O SpR Percivall Pott Rotation, London, UK
e-mail: cmail@nickaresti.com

M. Ramachandran, MBBS(Hons), MRCS, FRCS(Tr&Orth)
Consultant Orthopaedic and Trauma Surgeon,
Paediatric and Young Adult Orthopaedic Unit,
The Royal London and Barts
and The London Children's Hospitals,
Barts Health NHS Trust, London, UK
e-mail: manojorthopod@gmail.com

N.A. Aresti et al. (eds.), *Paediatric Orthopaedic Trauma in Clinical Practice*, In Clinical Practice,
DOI 10.1007/978-1-4471-6756-3_5,
© Springer-Verlag London Ltd. 2015

5.2   Epidemiology

Pelvic fractures in children are rare, accounting for between 2.4 and 7.5% of all childhood fractures. Mortality rates following pelvic fractures are approximately 6% and therefore considerably lower than mortality rates for adult pelvic fractures. Rates of pelvic fractures amongst children do not vary considerably with age. Pelvic avulsion fractures are most common amongst children engaged in sporting activities. Acetabular fractures account for 6–17% of pelvic fractures. Hip fractures are account for less than 1% of all childhood fractures.

5.3   Anatomical Considerations

5.3.1   Pelvis

A child's pelvis is malleable and the increased elasticity means more energy can be absorbed by cartilaginous structures. The pubic symphisis and sacroiliac joints are more elastic and therefore:

- More displacement is possible before permanent diastasis.
- A single fracture of the ring may occur as opposed to the double fracture seen in adults.

Avulsion fractures may occur through or near an apophysis. The immaturity of the hip and pelvis means that disruption of the epiphyseal or apophyseal growth plates may cause growth disturbance. This may occur following disruption to the triradiate cartilage, although it is more commonly seen with femoral epiphyseal disruption. Conversely the fractured immature pelvis has a good remodelling potential.

- Ossification centres:
  - Primary:
    - Triradiate cartilage fuses ≈ 12–14 years.
    - Pubic rami fuse ≈ 6–7 years.

- Secondary, so as not to confuse with avulsion fractures:

  - Iliac crest – first seen at 13–15. Fuses ≈ 17.
  - Ischium – first seen at 15–17. Fuses ≈ 19–25.
  - AIIS – first seen at 14. Fuses ≈ 16.

- Acetabular, so as not to confuse with avulsion fractures or loose bodies in hip:

  - Os acetabuli – starts to develop at 8. Fuses with pubis ≈ 18.
  - Acetabular epiphysis – starts to develop at 8. Fuses with ilium ≈ 18.
  - Secondary centre of ischium– starts to develop at 9. Fuses with pubis ≈ 17.

5.3.2 Hip

Ossification centers of the hip are as follows:

- Upper/capital femoral epiphysis begins to ossify at 4–6 months.
  - It accounts for only 13% of growth of the entire leg.
- Trochanteric ossification centres appear at 4 years.
- Fusion of the proximal femoral and trochanteric physes occurs at 14 in girls and 16 in boys.

Up until the age of 4, the femoral head is supplied by traversing metaphyseal vessels from the medial and lateral circumflex arteries. After the age of 4, as with adults, the lateral epiphyseal vessels supply the femoral head through posterosuperior and posteroinferior branches of the medial circumflex femoral artery. The artery of the ligamentum teres is of little importance. The hip is enclosed in a thick capsule. A haemarthrosis may occlude the vessels supplying the femoral head due to increased intra-articular pressure.

5.4   Pelvic Fractures

5.4.1   Fracture Classification

There are several classification systems for paediatric pelvic fractures however none have been able to conclusively correlate the mechanisms, patterns of injury, prognosis and treatment options with the varying skeletal maturity. Despite this, many recent studies have classified fractures based on the Torode and Zieg or Tile and Pennal classifications.

Silber and Flynn categorised 133 child pelvic fractures into immature (Risser 0 and all physes open) and mature (closed triradiate cartilage). They demonstrated that immature pelvic fractures rarely need operative intervention.

It is therefore recommended that fractures are classified as:

- Mature or immature.
- Stable or unstable.

  - In an immature pelvis, attention should be initially focused on concomitant injuries as the child's pelvis is unlikely to require operative intervention.
  - In a mature pelvis, fractures should be treated as per adult pathways and protocols.

Torode and Zieg

1. Avulsion fractures.
2. Iliac wing fractures.

   (a) Separation of the iliac apophysis.
   (b) Fracture of the bony iliac wing.

3. Simple ring fractures.

   (a) Fractures of the pubis and disruption of the pubic symphysis.
   (b) Fractures involving the acetabulum, without a concomitant ring fracture.

4. Fractures producing an unstable segment (ring disruption fracture).

   (a) "Straddle" fractures, characterized by bilateral inferior and superior pubic rami fractures.
   (b) Fractures involving the anterior pubic rami or pubic symphysis and the posterior elements (e.g. sacroiliac joint, sacral ala).
   (c) Fractures that create an unstable segment between the anterior ring of the pelvis and the acetabulum (Figs. 5.1).

Tile and Pennal

A. Stable fractures.

   A1. Avulsion fractures.
   A2. Undisplaced pelvic ring or iliac wing fractures.
   A3. Transverse fractures of the sacrum and coccyx.

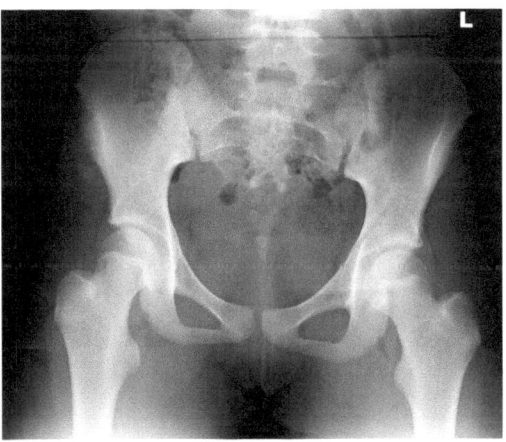

FIGURE 5.1 An X-ray showing an avulsion fracture of the right anterior superior iliac spine

B. Partially unstable fractures.

    B1. Open book fractures.
    B2. Lateral compression injuries (includes triradiate injury).
    B3. Bilateral type B injuries.

C. Unstable fractures of the pelvic ring.

    C1. Unilateral fractures.

        C1-1. Fractures of the ilium.
        C1-2. Dislocation or fracture-dislocation of the sacroiliac joint.
        C1-3. Fractures of the sacrum.

    C2. C2. Bilateral fractures, one type B, one type C.
    C3. Bilateral type C fractures (Figs. 5.2, 5.3, and 5.4).

5.4.2   Diagnosis

Avulsion fractures present with localized tenderness and swelling over the fracture site. There is typically a progressive

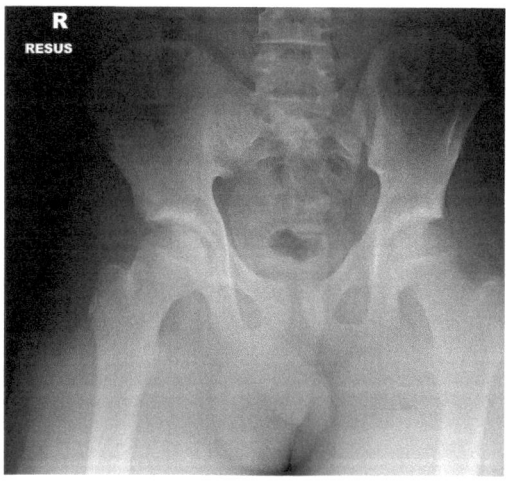

FIGURE 5.2 Fractures of the left inferior and superior pubic ramus, left sacral alar and widening of the sacral-iliac joints bilaterally

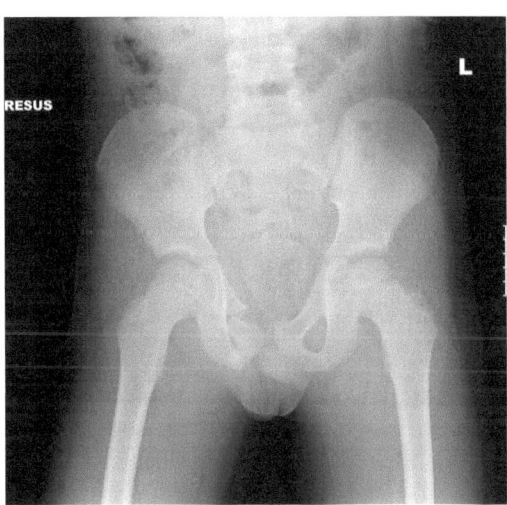

FIGURE 5.3 X-ray showing an undisplaced fracture of the right inferior sacral alar extending into the sacroiliac joint. There is a displaced fracture of the right inferior pubic ramus and a minimally displaced fracture of the right superior pubic ramus. There is also a minimally displaced fracture involving the left superior pubic rami

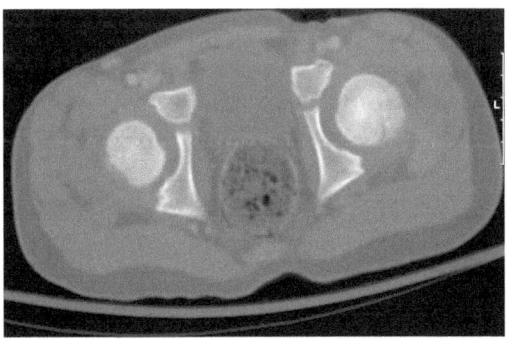

FIGURE 5.4 This is a CT scan of the same patient as Fig. 5.3. It demonstrates the left superior pubic fracture, which extends to involve the left acetabulum

limitation to range of motion. Patients with ischial avulsions experience pain on hip flexion and knee extension, with exaggeration of the pain on hip abduction.

In traumatic pelvic fractures, a full clinical evaluation of a child is necessary with adherence to ATLS protocols. A primary survey and examinations of the chest, abdomen and genitourinary systems should be performed prior to the pelvis. This should include a rectal examination.

When examining the pelvis:

- Inspect for lacerations, constusions, haematomas and ecchymosis.
- Examine for tenderness, stability and crepitus.
- Examine the range of motion of the hip.
- Perform a full distal neurological examination.
- A painful Trendelenburg sign may suggest an iliac wing fracture (due to abductor muscle contraction).

When assessing a patient following a traumatic episode, establish the maturity of the pelvis as early as possible, by obtaining a good quality AP X-ray of the pelvis during the trauma series. Haemodynamic instability is most likely due to a cardiac or abdominal cause – look elsewhere first.

5.4.3   Imaging

In patients who have sustained a significant trauma, imaging should be preceded by an initial clinical assessment and stabilization of the pelvis where necessary.

- In an acute setting, an AP X-ray of the pelvis suffices.
- This should be performed as part of the trauma series once the patient is stabilized.
- Inlet and outlet view X-rays of the pelvis may be deferred.
- A CT scan of the pelvis is indicated if there is:

    - Doubt with regards to possible injuries.
    - A plan to perform surgery.

5.4.4 Treatment

The treatment of pelvic and hip fractures depends on the exact injury. The table below summarises the likely mechanism of injury and recommended treatment for the various types of injuries seen.

Fracture	Likely mechanism of injury	Treatment
Avulsion	Ischial tuberosity – Gymnastics ASIS/AIIS – Football Iliac apophysitis – Long distance running	Most do well with conservative management, partial weight bearing for ≥ 2 weeks and extremity positioning Indications for surgery are chronic pain and acute fractures of >1–2 cm
Unilateral single or double rami fractures	High energy trauma Chronic repetitive stress (stress fractures to single ramus)	Bed rest Gradual weight bearing as pain allows
Wing of ilium (Duverney fracture)	Direct trauma	Bed rest in a comfortable position, usually with the leg abducted
Coccyx	Direct trauma	Restriction of activities. Doughnut cushion for 4–6 weeks.

(continued)

Fracture	Likely mechanism of injury	Treatment
Fracture near, or subluxation of, pubic symphysis	High energy trauma. Usually associated with posterior structures.	Isolated fractures or subluxation –side lying bed rest. Unilateral Buck's traction for pain. Reduction required if: Diastasis ≥ 2.5 cm Rotational deformity $> 15°$
Fracture near, or subluxation of, sacroiliac joint	High energy trauma, especially where there are injuries to posterior structures	Isolated injuries can be treated with bed rest and guarded weight bearing

Unstable fracture patterns

Bilateral superior & inferior pubic rami (straddle fractures)	Fall while straddling a hard object Lateral compression of pelvis Results in floating fragment	Commonly associated with bladder/urethral injury Inlet views show fractures most accurately Should heal regardless of amount of displacement Supine bed rest in semi-Fowler position If lateral compression fracture avoid lateral decubitus postion

Fracture	Likely mechanism of injury	Treatment
Complex fracture patterns, including posterior arch (posterior to acetabulum), bilateral anterior and posterior (most likely to cause haemorrhage)	Anteroposterior compression Lateral compression Indirect transmitted forces through femur with hip abducted and extended	CT and inlet views to assess degree of displacement Minimal displacement – bed rest in lateral recumbent position Severe lateral displacement – closed manipulation in lateral decubitus postion Cephalad displacement – skeletal traction (small children)

5.4.5   Indications for Surgery

Surgery for pelvic fractures in children is rarely indicated for a variety of reasons:

- Exsanguination is rare.
- Periosteum is thick and stabilizes fractures.
- Significant remodelling is possible.
- Nonunion is rare.
- There are good long-term morbidity rates.

As a result there are no clear-cut indications for surgery. Relative indictations indications include:

- Haemorrhage.
- Open fractures.
- To allow mobility.
- To facilitate nursing.
- To minimize growth disruption.
- To prevent deformity in fractures which are unlikely to remodel.
- To improve the overall care in polytrauma patients.

5.5   Acetabular Fractures

5.5.1   Fracture Classification

Several classification systems exist. The AO classification describes 3 types of fractures:

- A – partial articular, involving one of the two columns.
- B – partial articular, involving a transverse component.
- C – complete articular fractures, involving both columns.

5.5.2   Diagnosis

Acetabular fractures can be as a result of high or low energy trauma. A full clinical evaluation is required as described above. Furthermore, acetabular fractures are often associated with other pelvic injuries, which should be looked for.

5.5.3   Imaging

- AP X-rays may not show the extent of an acetabular fracture.
- Inlet, outlet and Judet views (45° oblique) may be necessary.
- CT scan allows further evaluation and assessment of any fragments within the acetabulum.
- Some advocate the use of MRI scans to assess the true size of cartilaginous structures.

5.5.4   Treatment and Indications for Surgery

- Aims are to restore joint congruity and hip stability.
- For non- or minimally displaced fractures (<1 mm), bed rest or non weight bearing ambulation may be indicated.
- For fractures displaced <2 mm, skeletal traction with a distal femoral traction pin may be used.

- Fractures >2 mm are likely to require ORIF.
- Few groups advocate surgery of all acetabular fractures, including the completion of partial fractures, and pelvic osteotomies where necessary.
- Postoperative application of a hip spica may be necessary for 6 weeks in the very young.

5.5.5   Complications of Pelvic and Acetabular Fractures

- Neurovascular injury.
- Skeletal deformity.
- Pelvic asymmetry.
- Premature arthritis.
- Premature triradiate cartilage closure.
- Hypertrophic myositis ossificans – acetabular fractures.
- Chronic long-term back pain.

5.6   Hip Fractures

Hip fractures in children differ considerably from the typical adult fragility fractures, requiring a considerable force. Mechanisms of injury include:

- Direct trauma.
- Axial loading.
- Torsion.
- Hyperabduction.

5.6.1   Fracture Classification

Delbet's classification is generally used as it is simple, allows accurate description and gives an indication of prognosis and management. It describes 4 categories and excludes subtrochanteric fractures.

Delbet's Paediatric Hip Fracture Classification

- Type I – transphyseal.
  - Type IA – without femoral head displacement.
  - Type IB – with femoral head displacement from the acetabulum.
- Type II – transcervical.
- Type III – cervicotrochanteric.
- Type IV – intertrochanteric.

5.6.1.1 Type I (Transphyseal)

- High-energy trauma, occasionally child birth.
- Approximately half are associated with dislocation of the upper femoral epiphysis, which leads to premature physeal closure and AVN in almost all cases.

5.6.1.2 Type II (Transcervical)

- Most common type.
- Risk of AVN related to degree of displacement.

5.6.1.3 Type III (Cervicotrochanteric)

- Second most common.
- Risk of AVN related to degree of displacement at the time of injury.
- Premature physeal closure occurs in 25% and coxa vara in 14% of cases.
- Displaced type III fractures have similar complications to type II fractures.
- Undisplaced type III fractures have few complications.

5.6.1.4 Type IV (Intertrochanteric)

- Have low complication rates (Fig. 5.5).

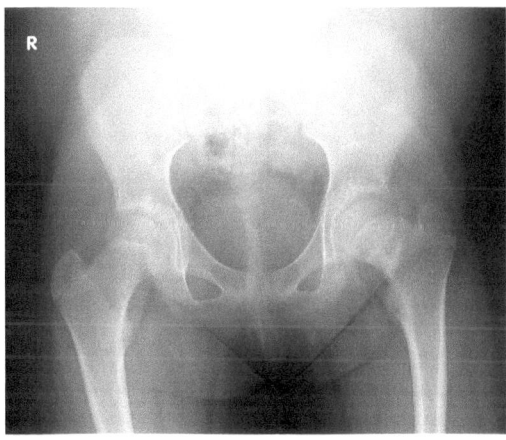

FIGURE 5.5 An impacted fracture of the left femoral neck

5.6.2 Diagnosis

As with pelvic fractures, hip fractures are most commonly as a result of high energy trauma. Patients should be evaluated as per ATLS and local protocols.

Patients may present similarly to adults with a painful hip, which is shortened and externally rotated, and inability to weight bear. Infants may hold their hip in flexion, abduction and external rotation. Undisplaced fractures of the femoral neck may be harder to detect, with children able to weight bear but with pain at the extremes of movement, in particular internal rotation.

5.6.3 Imaging

An AP X-ray will detect most fractures. The ideal position is in extension and as much internal rotation as pain allows. An 'on table' lateral X-ray should be performed instead of a frog leg lateral to avoid further displacement. MRI scans may be used to detect fractures that have not been picked up on X-ray within the first 24 h following an injury. A bone scan is an alternative to an MRI, being able to detect fractures around 48 h after injury.

5.6.4 Treatment

Treatment is based on fracture classification and age.

Age	Displacement	Treatment
Type I		
<2	Undisplaced/minimally displaced	Hip spica cast immobilization, in neutral and mild abduction
	Displaced	Closed reduction where possible +/− percutaneous pin fixation. Younger children with K-wires, older children with cannulated screws.
>2	Undisplaced/minimally displaced	
	Displaced	ORIF
Type II and III		
<5	Undisplaced/minimally displaced	Hip spica (for type II only) and/or internal fixation with cannulated screws
	Displaced	Closed reduction with longitudinal traction, abduction and internal rotation where necessary, or open reduction followed by cannulated screw fixation.
>5	Undisplaced/minimally displaced	
	Displaced	
Type IV		
<3	Undisplaced/minimally displaced	Hip spica
	Displaced	Closed reduction (with traction and internal rotation) or internal reduction, and hip spica
>3	Undisplaced/minimally displaced	ORIF with paediatric hip screw
	Displaced	

- Surgery within 24 hours will reduce the risk of complications.
- A haemarthrosis may lead to compromise of the blood supply to the femoral head.
- Early drainage of a haemarthrosis is advised.

5.6.5   Complications

Complications of hip fractures are frequent and significant. Because the hip is developing in children, deformities can progress with age. Complications include:

- Avascular necrosis (AVN):
    - Most common and perhaps most serious.
    - Related to initial displacement.
    - Caused by direct vessel damage or haemarthrosis induced occlusion of vessels through an increase in intra-articular pressure.
    - Most at risk fracture patterns are: type IB, type II and type III.
    - Ratliff described 3 types of AVN:

        - Type I: whole head.
        - Type II: partial head.
        - Type III: femoral neck.

    - X-ray changes may appear as early as 6 weeks.
    - MRI may show AVN within a few days of injury. If an MRI does not show AVN by 6 weeks, it is unlikely to develop.
    - Signs and symptoms appear between 1 and 2 years.
    - Early operative intervention (within 24 h) and early drainage of haemarthrosis has been shown to lower rates of AVN.

- Coxa vara.

    - This may be secondary to AVN, non-union, premature physeal closing or combinations of these pathologies.

- Premature physeal closure.
  - Most common in patients with type II and III fractures.
  - The risk is increased when the physis is crossed by fixation devices.

- Nonunion.

  - Generally due to failure to attain proper anatomical alignment.
  - Mainly type II and III fractures – rarely seen after type I or IV fractures.
  - Pain should be gone and bridging bone seen by 3 months.
  - Nonunion should be treated as soon as possible by operative intervention.

5.7   Synopsis

Pelvic fractures in children are a result of a high energy or violent trauma. The pelvic fracture is unlikely to cause mortality and attention should initially be focused on head, chest and abdominal injuries. The immature and mature pelvis should be distinguished. Mature pelvic fractures and acetabular fractures are most likely to need operative intervention.

Key References

Ismail N, Bellemare JF, Mollitt DL, DiScala C, Koeppel B, Tepas 3rd JJ. Death from pelvic fracture: children are different. J Pediatr Surg. 1996;31(1):82–5.

Silber JS, Flynn JM. Changing patterns of pediatric pelvic fractures with skeletal maturation: implications for classification and management. J Pediatr Orthop. 2002;22(1):22–6.

Ratliff AH. Fractures of the neck of the femur in children. J Bone Joint Surg Br. 1962;44-B:528–42.

Chapter 6
Paediatric Femoral Fractures

John Stammers and Matthew Barry

6.1 Epidemiology

Femur fractures are the third most common paediatric fracture requiring admission (after tibia and forearm); the incidence is reported as between 20 and 50 per 100,000 children, per year. There is a bimodal distribution - early childhood and mid-adolescence, with an equal sex distribution during the early childhood peak where the common mechanism is falls. In mid-adolescents, due to an increased risk from sports and motor vehicle collisions, males are more commonly affected.

The reported rate of non-accidental injury in femoral fractures under five is quoted between 10 and 40% with an increased likelihood in non-walkers.

J. Stammers, MBBS, BSc (Hons), MRCS (✉)
T&O SpR Royal London Rotation, London, UK
e-mail: john.stammers@nhs.net

M. Barry, MS, FRCS (Orth)
Consultant Orthopaedic and Trauma Surgeon,
Paediatric and Young Adult Orthopaedic Unit,
The Royal London and Barts and The London Children's Hospitals,
Barts Health NHS Trust, London, UK

N.A. Aresti et al. (eds.), *Paediatric Orthopaedic Trauma in Clinical Practice*, In Clinical Practice,
DOI 10.1007/978-1-4471-6756-3_6,
© Springer-Verlag London Ltd. 2015

6.2   Fracture Classification

Fractures can be classified using the following descriptive terms:

- Location: proximal, middle, distal third.
- Pattern: spiral, oblique, transverse, multifragmentary.
- Soft tissue: closed/open Anderson-Gustilo.
- Displacement: translation, angulation, rotation, impaction, distraction.

The AO system is used to classify diaphyseal fractures, but although comprehensive, it is rarely used in clinical practice.

6.3   Diagnosis

Femoral fractures typically present following a history of trauma and symptoms which include:

- Thigh pain.
- Inability to weight-bear.
- Reluctance to move the leg.

The mechanism of injury should be ascertained to determine the energy of the mechanism, the likelihood of associated injuries, and to rule out NAI.

When examining a patient with a femoral fracture:

- Inspect for swelling, lacerations, contusions, haematoma and ecchymosis.
- Palpate for tenderness and pulsatile swelling.
- Perform a full distal neurovascular examination.
- Examine the knee for swelling, deformity and instability (4% ipsilateral knee injury associated paediatric femoral fracture).
- In high-energy trauma perform a thorough secondary survey as other injuries can be missed in the presence of this distracting injury.
- If NAI is suspected, inspect for patterns of bruising, burns, previous fractures and head trauma.

AP and lateral radiographs of the femur should be taken. Following high-energy injuries, a trauma series should be performed, and where NAI is suspected, a skeletal survey should be requested.

6.4   Treatment

Various treatment options exist, depending on age and the characteristics of the fracture. Non operative options include (Table 6.1):

- Traction.
    - Pavlik harness for babies < 6 months of age.
    - Skin traction.
    - Skeletal traction (Fig. 6.1).

- Immediate hip spica casting.
- Delayed hip spica casting after 10–14 days.

Deciding on the type of fixation also varies with age. An algorithm to help decide accordingly is summarised in Table 6.2. Options include:

- Flexible intramedullary nailing (Fig. 6.2).
- Compression plating.
- Submuscular plating (Fig. 6.3).
- Lateral entry locked intrameduallary nail.
- External fixation (Fig. 6.4).

Each technique has advantages and disadvantages and a number of factors need to be considered to determine the most appropriate option for managing paediatric femoral fractures (See Table 6.1).

6.5   Follow-Up

The age, fracture pattern, fixation choice, risk of growth arrest and malunion affect timing of follow-up. Close observation with weekly radiographs maybe necessary

FIGURE 6.1 Skeletal
traction with distal
femoral traction
pin

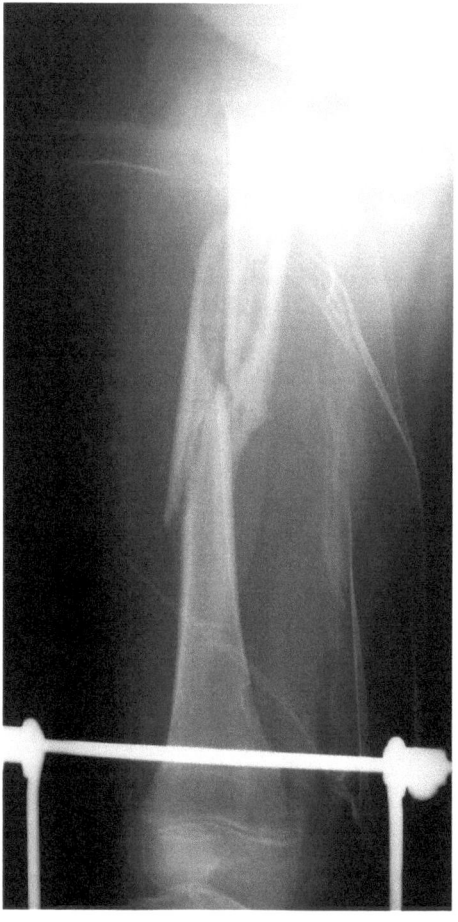

within the time period, so that any displacement is correctable. This is particularly relevant to conservatively managed fractures and unstable fracture patterns where additional splintage is used to complement fixation. Rigid fixation or uncomplicated fractures require wound review and radiographic assessment if it is intended to affect management, such as changing weight bearing status, removing metal work or contemplating treatment for symptomatic malunion.

FIGURE 6.2 Elastic intramedullary nails

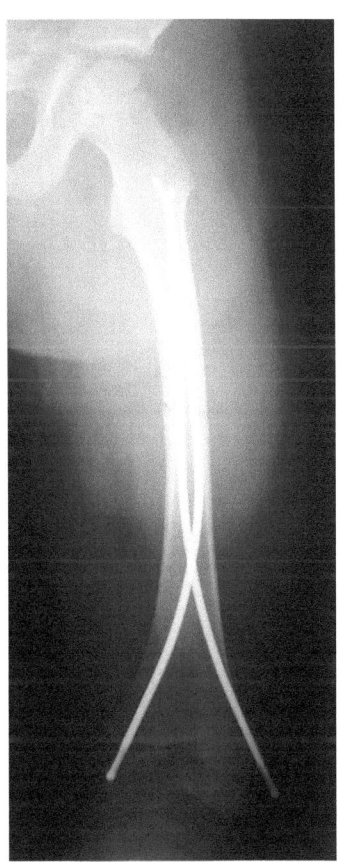

The fracture healing time varies with age:

Age	Approximate fracture healing time
0–6 months	3–4 weeks
6 months –2 years	4–6 weeks
2–12	3 months
12–18	3–6+ months

Many surgeons favour removing metalwork in children
primarily because of the difficulties encountered with late
removal (bone overgrowth of implant.) Other indications

FIGURE 6.3 Submuscular
plating

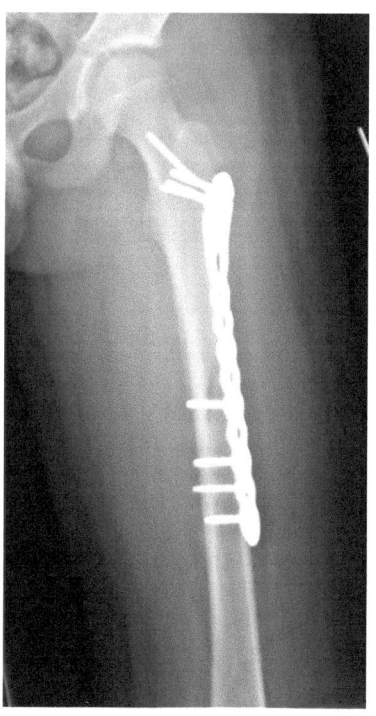

include a reduction in soft tissue irritation, a reduced range of movement of the knee and stress shielding.

Elastic nails are typically removed once the fracture has united but in units where removal is not routine, approximately 25% are removed due to soft tissue irritation. Complications with implant removal include refracture, infection, nerve injury and the inconvenience to parent and child of second surgery.

6.6   Complications

Various complications are possible following femoral fractures. These can be categorized as follows:

FIGURE 6.4 External fixation

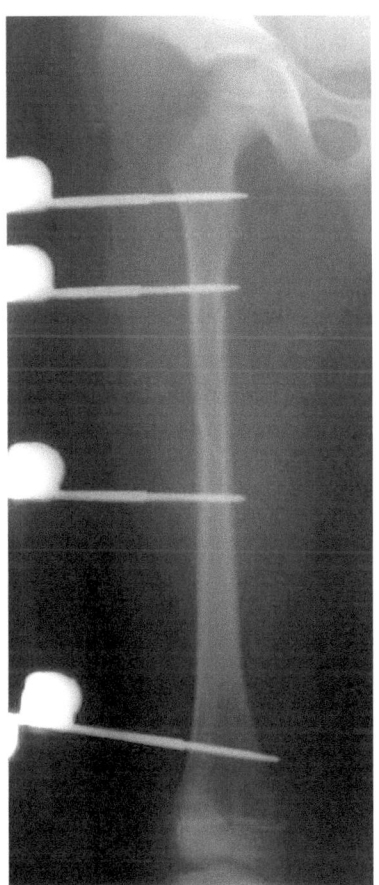

6.6.1   Skin

Pressure ulcers may occur following improper application of a spica cast. It is essential that any sharp edges are well padded and nearby skin checked regularly. Flexible elastic nails which may also cause irritation, if their ends are left too superficial.

TABLE 6.1 Management options, tips, advantages and disadvantages

Method	Age	Technical tips	Recommended	Contraindicated	Advantages	Disadvantages
Pavlik harness	<6 months	Ensure parents understand residual displacement will remodel	Proximal and middle third	Distal fractures, >6 months	Avoids skin irritation from spica cast	If >20° angulation deformities reliant on remodeling
Immediate spica casting	6 months–5 years	Close follow-up first 3 weeks, cast wedging to correct angulation deformity	Low energy, isolated fractures. Where telescope test results in less than 30 mm shortening	Multiple trauma, Obesity	Simple, proven history	Prolonged immobilization. Assessment of soft tissues and Skin loss Loss reduction
Traction and casting	6 months–5 years 5–10 years low energy	Traction pin inserted medial to lateral 90°–90° traction. Hip spica traction when no fracture site tenderness and radiographic evidence of callus (2-weeks) Traction weight 0.5 kg per year of life	Where shortening unacceptable for immediate casting. In increasing age or higher energy	Obesity Floating knee Head injury Polytrauma Distal fractures	Non-invasive.	Prolonged hospital stay. Outdated with internal fixation techniques

Flexible nailing	5–12	Nail diameter 40% isthmus femur. Use nails of the same diameter	Transverse, short oblique fractures	Very proximal or very distal spiral fracture. Length unstable >49 kg	Early mobilization, avoids physis, reduced re-fracture.	Skin tip irritation, malunion/shortening in unstable fractures, proximal or distal fracture may require limited weight bearing or bracing
External fixation	5–16	Release TFL to allow knee movement	Severely injured, large soft tissue defect, wide area fracture comminution. If nailing or plating contraindicated	If amenable to nailing	Minimally invasive, quick, early weight bearing	Refracture following removal, pin site infection, knee stiffness, family and schooling stigma with frame. Delayed union. Construct too rigid for callus formation but reduction not stable enough for primary bone healing

(continued)

TABLE 6.1 (continued)

Method	Age	Technical tips	Recommended	Contraindicated	Advantages	Disadvantages
Compression plating	5–16		Early weight bearing, fractures not amenable to flexi or rigid nailing in presence head injury	Post traumatic hypovolaemia and head injury. Open contaminated wounds	Stable fixation, early mobilization, low rate malunion	Blood loss, infection, delayed union from periosteal stripping, scar
Submuscular plating	5–16		Length unstable fractures Proximal or distal fractures Femoral canal too narrow for rigid nailing		Stable fixation, early mobilization, low rate malunion, minimal soft tissue disruption	Technically demanding relies on indirect reduction techniques. Removal of metalwork can be difficult
Rigid trochanteric entry nailing	12+ (with caution in skeletally immature)	Nail entry point lateral to the tip of the greater trochanter associated with least rate AVN	Length unstable fractures Heavy patients >49 kg	Narrow femoral canal relative to nail diameter	Stable fixation, early mobilization	AVN, Trochanteric epiphysiodesis, femoral neck narrowing, coxa valga

6.6.2   Nerve Injury

The most commonly effected nerve is the peroneal nerve. Palsy may results from either prolonged traction, improper spica application or high energy trauma.

6.6.3   Fracture Malunion

Varus malalignment and ensuing malunion is perhaps the most common form of malunion, and is more common with cast management of proximal fractures. Initial valgus 3-point moulding can help neutralise this tendency. Similarly, cast wedging within the first 3–4 weeks can correct angulation deformities. Rotational malunion up to 30° is rarely symptomatic unless it exaggerates pre-existing deformity such as femoral anteversion.

Established deformities will remodel for up to 2 years, therefore any corrective osteotomy should be deferred within this period, unless the deformity is considered too great to correct physiologically. Acceptable displacements are summarised below:

TABLE 6.2 Maximum acceptable deformity for femoral shaft fracture with age

Age	Anterior/posterior arecurvatum/ procurvatum	Varus/ valgus	Rotationb	Length/ overriding
Birth 2	30	30	10°	15
2–5	20	15	10°	20
6–10	10	10	10°	15
11+	5	5	10°	10

aAngular deformity is tolerated proximally; remodelling is improved near the physis and for deformities in line with joint motion.
bExternal rotation is tolerated more than internal rotation.

6.6.4   Leg Length Discrepancy

If a patient presents with significant early shortening (>3 cm), the following options are possible:

- Re-reduce and recast in a 90°–90° cast.
- Returning the patient to traction remains an option if the fractures is less than 2 weeks old.
- Consider internal fixation to control shortening.

Overgrowth can occur secondary to fracture healing, due to increased blood flow into the limb. The amount of overgrowth however is unpredictable.

6.6.5   Compartment Syndrome

Compartment syndrome, a surgical emergency, is characterised by pain despite adequate analgesia and immobilization. If suspected, the following measures should be taken:

- Split spica.
- Release traction (overhead traction increases the risk due to a combination of stretching of the popliteal artery with hyperextension of the knee, the gravitational effect and compression from bandaging holding the traction).

If compartment syndrome is clinically suspected or if there are elevated compartment pressures, a fasciotomy should be performed in a timely manner.

6.6.6   Infection

Pin tract infection is a common complication of external fixators. On discharge, the child and parents should be educated in pin site care and have "frame nurse" contact for queries.

6.6.7   Growth Arrest

Misplaced external fixator pins or traction pins across physis may lead to growth disturbances (Fig. 6.5).

6.6.8   Avascular Necrosis (AVN)

Some series suggest that following rigid intra-medullary femoral nailing, rates of AVN are as high as 4%. By using a lateral entry point in antegrade nails, the risk may be reduced.

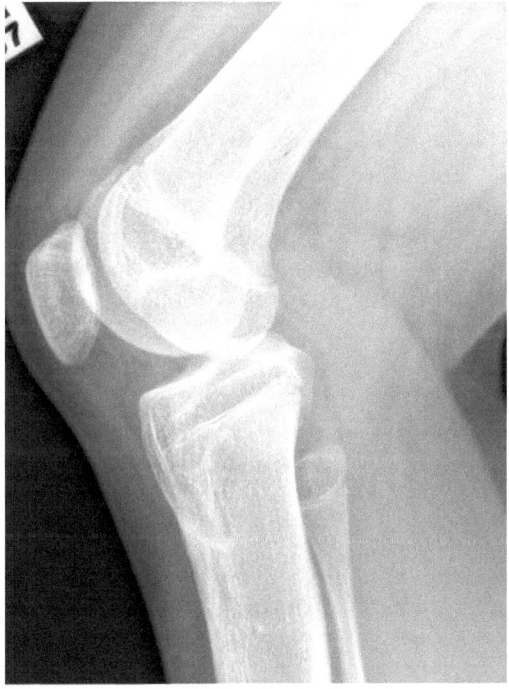

FIGURE 6.5 Apex posterior deformity proximal tibia after skeletal traction pin inserted through proximal tibia physis

6.6.9   Re-Fracture After Metalwork Removal

Given the risk of fracture, removal of elastic nails should be delayed for at least 6 months following fixation. Similarly, an external fixator should only be removed after 3 or more bridging cortices are visible on radiological follow-up.

6.6.10   Delayed Union or Non-union

Delayed and non-unions are rare in children but more common if managed with external fixators than other techniques.

6.7   Synopsis

Paediatric femoral fractures can be successfully managed by a number of techniques. Each option has advantages and disadvantages. It is important to consider patients age, weight, fracture position, stability, associated injuries and social issues in determining the most appropriate method to restore anatomy and function. Surgeons should be familiar with all potential treatment options or consider specialist opinion.

Key References

Kocher M, Sink E, Blasier R, et al. Treatment of pediatric diaphyseal femur fractures AAOS clinical practice guideline summary. J Am Acad Orthop Surg. 2009;17:718–25.

Flynn J, Luedtke L, Ganley T, et al. Comparison of titanium elastic nails with traction and a spica cast to treat femoral fractures in children. J Bone Joint Surg (Am). 2004;86-A(4):770–7.

MacNeil JA, Francis A, El-Hawary R. A systematic review of rigid, locked, intramedullary nail insertion sites and avascular necrosis of the femoral head in the skeletally immature. J Pediatr Orthop. 2011;31(4):377–80.

Blasier RD, Aronson J, Tursky EA. External fixation of pediatric femur fractures. J Pediatr Orthop. 1997;17(3):342–6.

Caird MS, Mueller KA, Puryear A, Farley FA. Compression plating of pediatric femoral shaft fractures. J Pediatr Orthop. 2003;23(4):448–52.

Li Y, Hedequist DJ. Submuscular plating of pediatric femur fracture. J Am Acad Orthop Surg. 2012;20(9):596–603.

MacNeil JA, Francis A, El-Hawary R. A systematic review of rigid, locked, intramedullary nail insertion sites and avascular necrosis of the femoral head in the skeletally immature. J Pediatr Orthop. 2011;31(4):377–80.

Chapter 7
Trauma of the Knee

Joanna Thomas and Claudia Maizen

7.1 Fractures About the Knee

Paediatric knee injuries differ from their adult counterparts both in terms of mechanism of injury and treatment options. Broadly speaking the injuries can be categorized by the affected bone and whether the fracture is intra-articular.

7.1.1 Distal Femoral Physeal Injuries

7.1.1.1 Introduction

Distal femoral physeal injuries represent around 2–5% of all physeal fractures. The distal femoral physis contributes 70% of growth in femur accounting for about 1.1 cm per year.

J. Thomas, MSc, FRCS (Tr&Orth) (✉)
T&O SpR Royal London Rotation, London, UK
e-mail: joanna.mckenna@me.com

C. Maizen, MD, (FRCS Orth)
Consultant Orthopaedic and Trauma Surgeon,
The Royal London and Barts and The London
Children's Hospitals, Barts Health, London, UK

N.A. Aresti et al. (eds.), *Paediatric Orthopaedic Trauma in Clinical Practice*, In Clinical Practice, DOI 10.1007/978-1-4471-6756-3_7, © Springer-Verlag London Ltd. 2015

It fuses with the metaphysis at approximately 14–16 years old in girls and 16–18 years old in boys. It can displace in the coronal and/or sagittal plane and can be associated with neurovascular injury.

7.1.1.2 Fracture Classification

Physeal injuries in the femur are classified as per the Salter-Harris classification system. The femoral physis undulates and contains mammillary processes therefore fractures involve many regions of the physis. This may contribute to the high incidence of growth arrest.

7.1.1.3 Diagnosis

Patients typically present with a history of a hyperextension or valgus injury. Injuries may follow a high-energy traumatic incident, similar to knee dislocation in adult. Examination reveals inability to weight bear, pain and swelling (often marked). In severe cases, deformity or tethering/puckering of the skin may be apparent.

Neurovascular examination is essential. The treating surgeon must have a low threshold for arranging angiography, particularly if there is a period of diminished pulses. Dislocated fractures should be managed with expedient reduction. Coronal plane (often valgus) injury may not be radiographically obvious so a high index of suspicion must remain.

7.1.1.4 Imaging

Stress radiographs or MRI scans may be useful in diagnosing undisplaced SH I fractures but repeat clinical examination is often adequate. Diagnosis is important to predict the possibility of growth arrest.

7.1.1.5 Treatment

Non-operative Treatment

- Undisplaced or minimally displaced fractures (usually SH I/II) are treated with a long-leg cast or hip spica, with the knee in slight flexion for 4–6 weeks.
- Any fracture that requires a GA for reduction usually requires internal fixation as late re-displacement can occur and increases the possibility of growth disturbance.

Indications for Surgery

- Anatomical reduction is best.
- >5° varus/valgus deformity as it is unlikely to remodel.
- Salter-Harris I or II fractures can usually be reduced closed but Salter-Harris III and IV fractures often require open reduction to ensure the articular surface is anatomical.

Methods of Surgical Fixation

- Closed reduction is achieved mainly by traction with minimal manipulation to reduce stresses on the growth plate.
- Salter-Harris I fractures should be stabilised by crossed K-wires that do not cross each other at the fracture site (see diagram). Wires should be placed with a single pass to minimise further damage to the growth plate.
- Salter-Harris II fractures can be stabilised by K-wire or screw fixation of the metaphyseal (Thurston-Holland) fragment if large enough, taking care to avoid the perichondrial ring of LaCroix. Fixation should be parallel to the physis and may be augmented with trans-epiphyseal K-wires.
- Salter-Harris III and IV fractures are treated with open, anatomical reduction and K-wire or screw fixation of the epiphysis with hardware placed parallel to physis (Fig. 7.1).
- A long leg cast should be applied for 4–6 weeks.

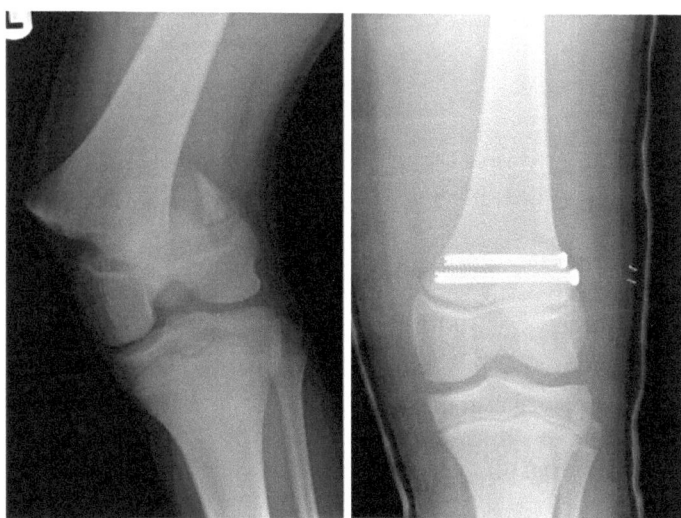

FIGURE 7.1 Radiographs of a distal femoral physeal injury and fixation using two parallel screws

7.1.1.6 Follow-Up

- K-wire pin sites should be checked at 1–2 weeks and the plaster cast replaced with a lightweight fibreglass cast.
- K-wires should be removed at 3–4 weeks, especially trans-epiphyseal crossed K-wires as they may be intra-articular and predispose to septic arthritis.
- All physeal fractures should be followed up for at least 1 year to look for a growth arrest.

7.1.1.7 Complications

These may be categorised as below:

- Immediate:
    - Neurovascular injury.
    - Malreduction.
    - Compartment syndrome.

- Early:
  - Re-displacement.
  - Infection.
- Late:
  - Growth arrest or angular deformity.
  - Limb length discrepancy.

7.1.1.8 Synopsis

These are uncommon injuries (2–5% of physeal fractures) that need to be considered with a high index of suspicion. They should be treated with anatomical reduction and internal fixation to minimise late angular deformity or growth arrest.

7.1.2   Proximal Tibial Physeal Injuries

7.1.2.1 Introduction

Proximal tibial physeal injuries are rare due to intrinsic stability as a result of the overlapping fibula, the anatomy of the tibial tubercle and the metaphyseal attachment of the medial collateral ligament (MCL). Considerable forces are required to separate the proximal tibial physis and therefore concomitant injuries are often seen. Vascular compromise is common due to the popliteal vessels being tethered in this region, and so compartment syndrome is an important consideration.

The proximal tibial physis contributes 60% toward the growth of the tibia, amounting to approximately 0.9 cm per year. Unlike distal femur fractures, proximal tibial physeal injuries rarely succumb to growth arrest after injury.

7.1.2.2 Fracture Classification

- The most common type of injury is a SH II, but towards end of growth the proximal tibial physis fuses from posterior to anterior, which may result in more SH III injuries.

7.1.2.3 Diagnosis

Patients present with a history of a direct force (such as following an RTA) or a hyperextension type injury. Examination reveals marked tenderness and swelling of the proximal tibia with a possible concavity at the level of the tibial tuberosity, if the metaphysis has been displaced posteriorly. As with all such knee injuries, always assess and document the neurovascular status, and observe the patient for a potential impending compartment syndrome.

7.1.2.4 Imaging

Begin with an AP and lateral of the knee, augmented with oblique films if the aforementioned views appear normal. Stress radiographs or CT/MRI may be helpful in diagnosis.

7.1.2.5 Treatment

Non-operative Treatment

- Undisplaced fractures may be treated in an above-knee backslab, then converted to a fibreglass cast with slight knee flexion for 6 weeks total.
- Always watch for compartment syndrome in the first few days.

Indications for Surgery

- Anatomical reduction is necessary for the best result. Anything short should be considered for surgical intervention.
- Even minimal posterior displacement of the metaphysis can occlude the popliteal artery, so thought must be given to treating posteriorly displaced fragments.
- Displaced SH I and II fractures can be treated with closed reduction, followed by trans-epiphyseal crossed K-wires passed from the metaphysis into the epiphysis. Whenever any physis is crossed, a single pass technique is advocated. The wires should not cross at the fracture site. Open

reduction may be required if the pes anserinus prevents closed reduction.

- Displaced SH III and IV fractures will often require opening to ensure anatomical reduction and placement of K-wires or screws horizontally into the epiphysis, and proximal and parallel to the physis.
- Fasciotomies are required if vascular compromise and compartment syndrome are identified.

7.1.2.6 Follow-Up

Backslabs should be removed and the wounds checked at 1–2 weeks. Full fibreglass casts should then be applied until the K-wires are removed at 3–4 weeks. The fibreglass above knee cast is discontinued at 6 weeks. Patients should be followed up for at least 1 year to observe for growth disturbance.

7.1.2.7 Complications

- Immediate:
    - Compartment syndrome.
    - Neurovascular compromise.
- Early:
    - Infection.
    - Malreduction.
- Late:
    - Angular deformity.
    - Growth arrest.
    - Limb length discrepancy.

7.1.2.8 Synopsis

A rare physeal injury but often associated with other injuries and vascular compromise or compartment syndrome. Anatomical reduction and internal fixation is required to prevent complication.

7.1.3   Tibial Tubercle Avulsion

7.1.3.1 Introduction

Avulsion of the tibial tubercle apophysis represents a SH III injury. It is most commonly seen in boys aged 12–16 years and associated with jumping sports due to sudden eccentric loading of the extensor mechanism. A large periosteal sleeve may be avulsed with the tubercle. Tibial tubercle avulsion should not be confused with Osgood-Schlatter disease which is a chronic condition of repeated micro-avulsion of the superficial tuberosity, not involving the apophysis.

7.1.3.2 Classification

The most widely used classification system was devised by Ogden. The system takes into account the two ossification centres in the proximal tibia: the primary ossification centre (proximal tibial physis) and the secondary ossification centre (tibial tubercle physis) (Fig. 7.2).

- Type I – fracture of the secondary ossification centre.
- Types II – fracutre propagates to the junction with the primary ossification centre.
- Type III – fracture crosses the primary ossification centre.
- Modification A: undisplaced.
- Modification B: displaced.

7.1.3.3 Diagnosis

Patients typically present following a jump or fall, followed by pain in the anterior aspect of their knee and inability to straight leg raise. Examination findings include swelling and tenderness over the tibial tubercle with the knee held in slight flexion. Some active knee extension may be present if retinacular fibres are intact. Patella alta may be noticed and the mobile bone fragment may be felt if it is large enough. Compartment syndrome has been reported.

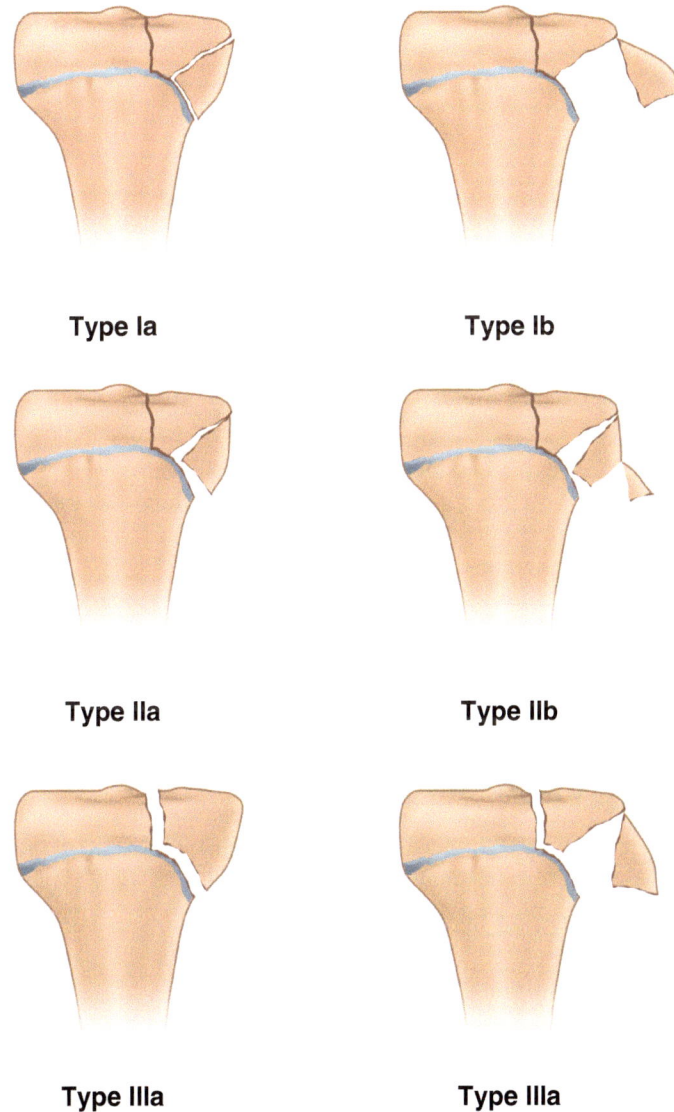

Type Ia

Type Ib

Type IIa

Type IIb

Type IIIa

Type IIIa

FIGURE 7.2 The Ogden classification

7.1.3.4 Imaging

Lateral knee radiographs will confirm the injury and show the amount of displacement. Look for patella alta and if necessary, compare to the non-injured side.

7.1.3.5 Treatment

- Type IA fractures (undisplaced) can be treated in a cylinder cast in full extension for 6 weeks.
- Type 1B, 2 and 3 fractures should be treated by open reduction and internal fixation. Cancellous or cortical screws are placed through the tuberosity fragment horizontally across the metaphysis. Large periosteal sleeves can be reattached using suture anchors if desired (Fig. 7.3).
- Type 3 fractures involve the articular surface and should therefore be reduced anatomically either by open or arthroscopic means.
- Type 3 fractures are associated with meniscal tears, which may need repair.

7.1.3.6 Follow-Up

Post-operatively, the limb is placed in full extension in a backslab. At 1–2 weeks the wound is inspected and the limb placed into a full fibreglass cylinder cast for total of 4–6 weeks post-op. Patients should be advised to avoid sports (especially jumping) for 4–6 months.

7.1.3.7 Complications

- Compartment syndrome.
- Prominent hardware, which usually requires removal.
- Growth arrest is normally not an issue as the injury tends to occur close to the end of growth.

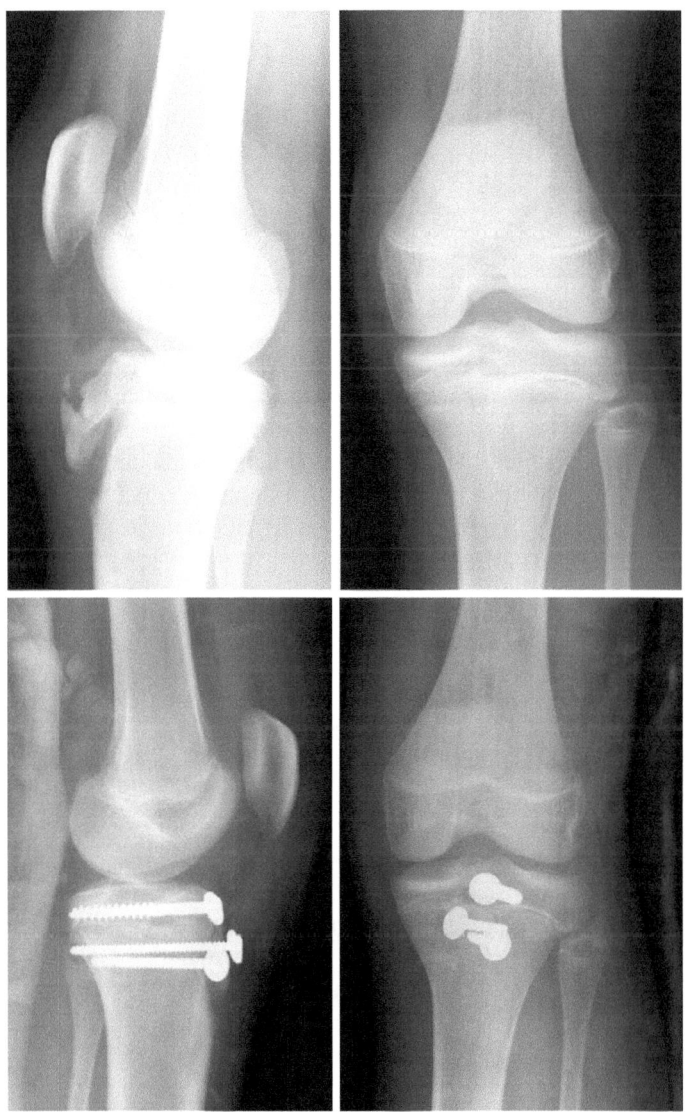

FIGURE 7.3 Pre and post op radiographs of a tibial tuberosity fracture

7.1.3.8 Synopsis

This is an injury of adolescence associated with jumping sports (often basket ballers) and often requires operative repair. Compartment syndrome is associated with these injuries.

7.1.4 Patella Sleeve Fractures

7.1.4.1 Introduction

Patella sleeve fractures are essentially an avulsion fracture of the distal (or rarely, proximal) pole of the patella, which pulls off a large amount of articular cartilage, disrupting the retinaculum. They occur in late childhood or early adolescence due to incomplete ossification of the patella, which commences between 3 and 6 years of age. The mechanism of injury is eccentric contraction of the quadriceps with the knee flexed, such as in jumping sports.

7.1.4.2 Imaging

Fractures are easily missed on plain radiographs. Instead patella alta or baja may be visible based on which sleeve fractures. MRI and USS may provide more information where the clinical picture necessitates further imaging (Fig. 7.4).

7.1.4.3 Classification

No useful classification system has been described but the amount of articular cartilage involved and the amount of displacement determines the need for surgery.

7.1.4.4 Diagnosis

Patients present with pain and swelling typically following a jumping injury or fall. An acute haemarthrosis is often present. A high or low riding patella and inability to straight leg raise would suggest an extensor retinaculum rupture although an extensor lag is common.

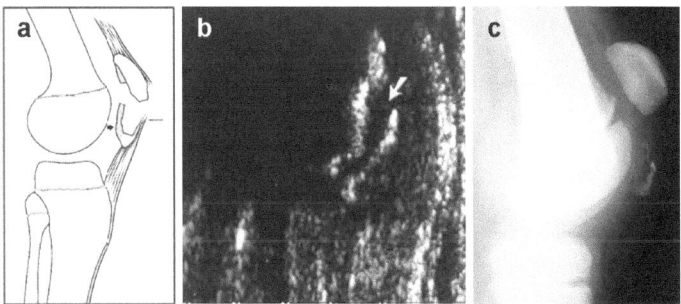

FIGURE 7.4 (**a**) Line drawing of a patellar sleeve fracture. (**b**) Ultrasound showing the periosteal sleeve. (**c**) Later radiograph of a missed case showing new bone formation in the sleeve, giving the appearance of a double patella (Figure and legend reprinted with permission from Benson et al. (2009) *Children's Orthopaedics and Fractures*, Springer)

7.1.4.5 Treatment

In fractures in which there is less than 2 mm of displacement and an intact extensor mechanism/retinaculum, treatment can remain non-operative, with a cylinder cast in extension.

Displaced fractures with disruption of the retinaculum should be treated with open anatomical reduction, internal fixation and retinacular repair. Tension band wiring (figure of eight wire) around two longitudinal K-wires provides rigid fixation. Alternatively, sutures (such as fibrewire) may be passed through longitudinal drill holes using a suture passer and tied over a bony bridge. The defect in the retinaculum is used to ensure the articular surface is reduced before it is securely repaired.

7.1.4.6 Follow-Up

Non-operatively treated fractures should remain in cast for 6–8 weeks. Those treated surgically should remain in a backslab in full extension for 1–2 weeks. Following a wound check, the patient should be placed into a fibreglass cylinder cast for a further 4 weeks. Patients should avoid jumping activities for 3–4 months and until knee flexion has been restored.

7.1.4.7 Complications

Ectopic bone formation and persistent limitation of knee flexion have been described. As the blood supply of the immature patella is from the distal pole, transient ischaemic changes can be seen, although they are uncommon.

7.1.4.8 Synopsis

Patella sleeve fractures occur in the adolescent knee as a result of eccentric contraction and are commonly missed. If treated expediently the outcome is good.

7.1.5 Tibial Spine Avulsion

7.1.5.1 Introduction

Tibial spine avulsion injuries are one of the commonest injuries of the knee in the paediatric population. They usually occur between the ages of 8 and 14. The mechanism of injury is similar to that of adult ACL ruptures, i.e. hyperextension or valgus rotational injury, such as a fall from a bicycle. Avulsion injuries rather than ACL ruptures occur as the ACL is stronger than the tibial intercondylar eminence. Coexistent ACL tear and meniscal/chondral injury may be present.

7.1.5.2 Fracture Classification

Meyers and McKeever first classified eminence fractures by dividing them into three types:

- Type I: undisplaced (slight elevation of anterior eminence).
- Type II: displaced fragment with posterior hinge.
- Type III: completely displaced fragment with or without rotation.

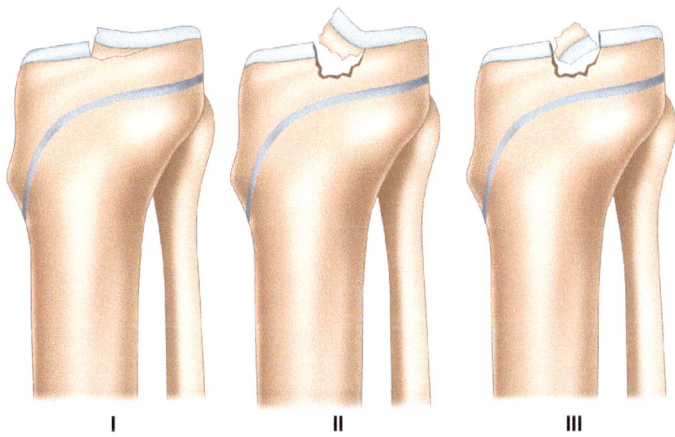

I   II   III

FIGURE 7.5 Meyers and McKeever classification

Comminution of the fragment in Type III injuries is common (Fig. 7.5).

7.1.5.3 Diagnosis

Patients present with a history of a fall from a bicycle/ motorbike, or following a twisting injury during pivoting sports. Examination reveals a haemarthrosis, pain on extremes of motion and a positive anterior drawer test or Lachman test (AP laxity may be difficult to detect due to haemarthrosis). The examination must include assessment of the collateral ligaments and the PCL.

7.1.5.4 Imaging

Plain radiographs may not reveal the fracture as the avulsion may include only non-ossified cartilage. An MRI scan will assist in the diagnosis and also enable diagnosis of meniscal or collateral ligament injuries.

7.1.5.5 Treatment

Type I injuries are treated non-operatively with 6 weeks in a long leg cast in 10–20° of flexion (ACL bundles are most relaxed in slight flexion). Type II and III injuries require operative reduction and fixation to prevent late instability.

Operative techniques vary and include arthroscopic or open surgery with screw or suture (fibrewire) fixation, the latter through two tunnels drilled using an ACL tibial guide and facilitated by the use of a suture passer with sutures tied over a bone bridge. Adequate reduction may be blocked by the medial meniscus or intermeniscal ligament, which sometimes requires the surgeon to convert an arthroscopic procedure into an open procedure.

Disadvantages of screw fixation include damage to the physis if caution is not taken to avoid it and the need for hardware removal.

7.1.5.6 Follow-Up

Post-operatively a long leg back slab or brace is applied in slight flexion and the wounds are checked in clinic at 1–2 weeks. At this stage the decision is made to continue immobilisation in a fibreglass cast for a further 2–3 weeks or commence early mobilisation. The authors preferred regime is early conversion to a brace with ROM 10–60° for 2–3 weeks then full ROM at 4–6 weeks post-op. This helps to prevent loss of terminal extension and does not risk disruption of a secure fixation.

7.1.5.7 Complications

Laxity can be caused by inadequate reduction or stretching/tear of the ACL at the time of injury. Malunion can be minimised by conversion to open procedure if visualisation is difficult through the arthroscope.

7.1.5.8 Synopsis

Tibial spine avulsion is caused by a hyperextension or twisting injury and if displaced requires operative reduction and fixation to prevent late laxity and instability.

7.1.6 Osteochondritis Dissecans (OCD)

7.1.6.1 Introduction

The name of this condition is a misnomer. OCD actually represents a defect in subchondral bone which results in partial or complete separation of a bone fragment and the overlying cartilage. Approximately 80% affect the lateral wall of the medial femoral condyle and are a common cause of intra-articular loose bodies.

The aetiology is not fully understood: OCD is thought to be caused by repetitive micro-trauma to the articular cartilage (although other theories exist) and should be distinguished from osteochondral fractures that are often seen affecting the patellofemoral joint after patellar dislocation.

7.1.6.2 Fracture Classification

There are a number of classification systems including those based on plain radiographs, MRI and arthroscopic examination. The important features, which affect prognosis, include skeletal maturity, size of the lesion and stability of the fragment.

The Pappas Classification divides patients into Juvenile, Adolescent and Adult forms of the condition. This helps predict prognosis.

The Guhl Classification is based on arthroscopic findings:

- Type 1: intact overlying cartilage.
- Type 2: early separation (stable flap).
- Type 3: partial detachment (unstable flap).
- Type 4: complete detachment.

7.1.6.3 Diagnosis

The history is often vague. Patients present with anterior knee pain, a limp and mechanical symptoms of the joint, including locking and "giving way". When mechanical symptoms are present a detached loose body within the knee should be looked for. Clinical examination is often normal.

7.1.6.4 Imaging

Radiographs, including skyline and tunnel views, demonstrate the defect. MRI scans further define the anatomy and allow assessment of size and stability. Perifocal sclerosis is a negative prognostic indicator.

7.1.6.5 Treatment

Juvenile forms of the disease have a good prognosis. When the physis is open, consider non-operative treatment, as up to 80% will heal. Non-weightbearing or partial weightbearing on crutches and avoidance of sport are the mainstay of treatment.

Adolescent forms (age 12–18 years old) have a variable prognosis and approximately 50% will heal with non-operative treatment. Adult forms (closed physis) of the disease have a poor prognosis and often require operative intervention. Unstable lesions require arthroscopic assessment and either fixation, removal and microfracture or drilling of the lesion, depending on the size and location. Large lesions may be considered suitable for cartilage regeneration techniques (e.g: autologous chondrocyte implantation).

7.1.6.6 Follow-Up

Follow-up depends on treatment modality but may include repeat MRI scan or arthroscopy to reassess the lesion. The development of new mechanical symptoms suggests detachment of the fragment.

7.1.6.7 Complications

Detachment of a large lesion will predispose to early arthritis.

7.1.6.8 Synopsis

Osteochondritis Dissecans (OCD) is an uncommon condition of the knee most commonly affecting the lateral wall of the medial femoral condyle. The treatment and prognosis are determined by the skeletal maturity of the patient and the size and stability of the lesion.

7.1.7   Anterior Cruciate Ligament (ACL) Rupture

7.1.7.1 Introduction

These injuries are rare yet they are becoming more commonly diagnosed. We are not sure as to whether the incidence itself is increasing or because diagnostic techniques are improving.

In the very young they are usually associated with a high-energy injury but in the older child and adolescent the mechanism is similar to adults (hyperextension or valgus rotational injury). The youngest reported ACL rupture is in a 3 year old but injuries sustained in children younger than 10 years of age are extremely rare.

The differential diagnosis for these injuries will include patella dislocation, collateral ligament injury and meniscal tear. Remember that congenital ACL deficiency can be associated with fibula hemimelia and proximal femoral focal deficiency (look for hypoplastic tibial spine).

7.1.7.2 Diagnosis

Patient's present with a history of hyperextension or a valgus rotational injury. Commonly swelling will appear over an hour or two. If swelling is more acute, then consider a fracture. Examination will reveal a haemarthrosis. It may be difficult to test for instability in the acute setting and repeat examination once the swelling has subsided is important.

7.1.7.3 Imaging

X-rays should be performed to exclude a fracture and to identify a lipohaemarthrosis (associated with a fracture). An MRI scan can be performed in the older child to assist in the diagnosis and treatment plan. Identification of a meniscal injury is important and will make early surgical intervention more likely. MRI in the younger child may require sedation and therefore the benefits and risks should be considered.

7.1.7.4 Treatment

Non-operative Treatment

Swelling reduction assisted by regular icing should be the mainstay of early treatment. Once the swelling has subsided and a full range of movement has been restored, a full assessment can be performed. Children who have regular instability and who will not refrain from sporting activities are likely to sustain meniscal tears whilst waiting for reconstruction. They have a poor prognosis.

Indications for Surgery

Many children will require surgical stabilisation at some stage and the age at presentation will help determine the treatment. If surgery is necessary, it is important to stabilise the knee without causing a growth arrest. In the very young child, this usually requires physeal sparing surgery but the early adolescent may be suitable for partial transphyseal or complete transphyseal reconstruction (as in the adult). There is increasing evidence that children over the age of 12–13 years (careful assessment of skeletal maturity is essential) do not experience significant growth disturbance with transphyseal ACL reconstruction as long as screws or bone-patella-bone grafts are not placed across the physis and hamstring grafts are used in preference.

7.1.7.5 Follow-Up

Regular follow-up is essential in the operately and non-operatively treated child. Those children who have had non-anatomical, physeal sparing surgery will likely require ACL reconstruction towards the end of skeletal maturity.

7.1.7.6 Complications

Non-operatively treated children are at high risk of sustaining meniscal injuries. Growth disturbance can be seen in children treated with transphyseal surgical stabilisation.

7.1.7.7 Synopsis

ACL ruptures are becoming increasingly common and are associated with poor prognosis in the younger child. Surgical reconstruction is often required and technique depends on the skeletal maturity of the patient.

7.1.8   Meniscal Injuries

7.1.8.1 Introduction

Meniscal injures are less commonly seen than in the adult but they have a higher incidence with ligament injuries (ACL) and subsequent instability. Injuries are more often associated with a discoid meniscus. 1% of children are estimated to have a discoid lateral meniscus, some presenting with 'snapping knee syndrome'.

7.1.8.2 Classification

Meniscal tears can be classified as to their orientation, e.g. they may be longitudinal, vertical or peripheral.

A discoid meniscus can be classified using the Watanabe classification:

- Type 1: complete (Stable).
- Type 2: incomplete (Stable).
- Type 3: unstable – crescent shape but absent meniscotibial ligaments = Wrisberg variant.

7.1.8.3 Diagnosis and Radiography

History and examination are important diagnostic tools. Plain radiography may show evidence of a discoid meniscus, namely a widened lateral joint line and cupping of the lateral plateau. False positive results for meniscal tear can be seen on MRI due to the increased peripheral vascularity of the meniscus. Clinical diagnosis should be made by careful examination.

7.1.8.4 Treatment

Symptomatic meniscal tears should be treated with an arthroscopic repair, if at all possible. An asymptomatic discoid meniscus or painless 'snapping knee syndrome' should be left untreated. If a discoid meniscus is torn, the treating surgeon should consider a meniscoplasty (saucerisation) and/or stabilisation to the capsule (Wrisberg variant).

7.1.8.5 Follow-Up

Some would advocate repeat arthroscopy 6 months after meniscal repair to assess healing.

7.1.8.6 Complications

Menisectomy in the child or adolescent will predispose to osteoarthritis in adulthood so preservation of meniscal tissue is a priority.

7.1.8.7 Synopsis

Meniscal tears are often associated with ligament injuries or a discoid meniscus. Preservation of meniscal tissue is a priority but consider meniscoplasty in a torn discoid meniscus.

Chapter 8
Paediatric Tibial Fractures

Kalpesh R. Vaghela and Matthew Barry

8.1 Introduction

Tibial fractures are amongst the most common injuries encountered in paediatric trauma. They include a spectrum from low energy toddler's (diaphyseal) fractures to high-energy open tibial fractures. In addition to this, there are rarer tibial injuries with potential significant complications. This chapter utilises an anatomic approach (proximal, diaphyseal, and distal) to classify paediatric tibial fractures and discusses their diagnosis, classification, management, and complications.

8.2 Epidemiology

Tibial fractures constitute 15% of all paediatric fractures. The diaphysis is involved in 39% of cases, with a fibula fracture in 30% of cases. Boys are affected more than girls with a peak

K.R. Vaghela, MBBS BSc MRCS DipMedEd (✉)
T&O SpR Percivall Pott Rotation, London, UK
e-mail: kalpeshrvaghela@gmail.com

M. Barry, MS, FRCS (Orth)
Consultant Orthopaedic and Trauma Surgeon,
Paediatric and Young Adult Orthopaedic Unit,
The Royal London and Barts and The London Children's Hospitals,
Barts Health NHS Trust, London, UK

N.A. Aresti et al. (eds.), *Paediatric Orthopaedic Trauma
in Clinical Practice*, In Clinical Practice,
DOI 10.1007/978-1-4471-6756-3_8,
© Springer-Verlag London Ltd. 2015

incidence of around 8 years. Proximal tibial fractures are rare accounting for less than 1%.

8.3   Anatomical Considerations

- The tibia is surrounded by the four muscle compartments of the leg but is exposed anteromedially rendering it susceptible to injury and open fractures. There is also limited healing potential at this site with large skin defects requiring soft tissue coverage by the plastic surgeons.
- It is closely related to the fibula to which it is bound by a strong interosseous membrane.
- There is a small amount of proximal/distal translation and internal/external rotation at the proximal and distal tibio-fibular joints.

8.4   Ossification Centres

8.4.1   Proximal Tibial Physis (Fig. 8.1)

- Growth contribution – 6 mm/year.
- The proximal tibial physis contributes approximately 55% of the final tibial length, and 25% of the whole length of the limb..
- The epiphyseal ossification centre appears at 1–3 months.
- Primary ossification centre – the center of the ossification reaches the tibial eminence in late childhood. The centre slowly enlarges to the secondary centre from posterior to anterior.
- Secondary ossification centre.

    - Cartilaginous stage is from 8 to 10 years.
    - Apophyseal stage – distal tibial tuberosity ossification appears at 8–14 years of age.
    - Epiphyseal stage – ossification centre of the tubercle and proximal tibial epiphysis fuse at 17 years of age.

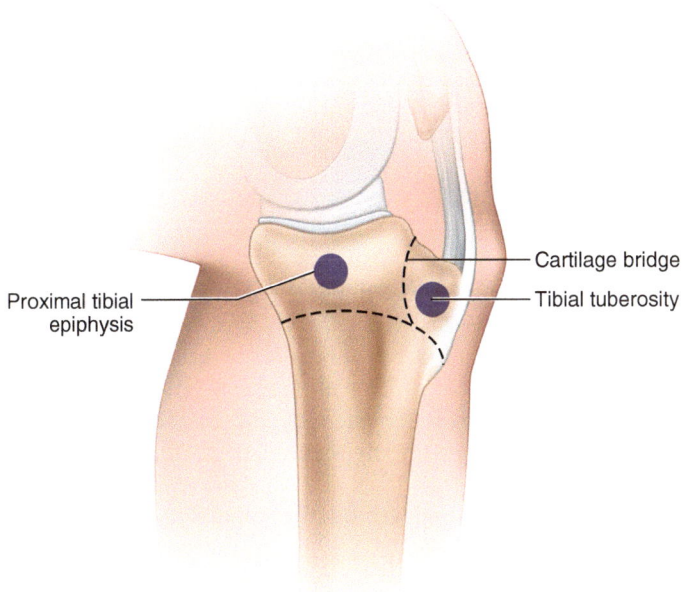

FIGURE 8.1 Proximal tibia physis anatomy

  – Bony stage – physis closes between tuberosity and metaphysis.
• The physis of tuberosity closes in girls at 13-5 years and boys at 15-19 years.

8.4.2   Diaphyseal Physis

• Ossifies at 7 weeks of gestation and extends proximally and distally to meet the other tibial physes.

8.4.3 Distal Tibial Physis

- Growth contribution – 5 mm/year.
- Closure of the physis follows a predictable pattern. From central to medial, then progresses laterally. The anterolateral area closes last at around 14 years of age. See diagram below (Fig. 8.2).

8.5 Blood Supply

- The thick periosteum provides a significant proportion of the blood supply to the tibia.
- Proximal tibia – this is supplied by a rich extraosseous supply from the popliteal artery, anterior tibial artery (ATA) laterally, and the posterior tibial artery (PTA) medially.
- Diaphysis – this is supplied by the nutrient artery, and so is a considerably hypovascular region, particularly posteriorly.
- Distal tibia – supplied by the medial ATA and PTA anastomosis.

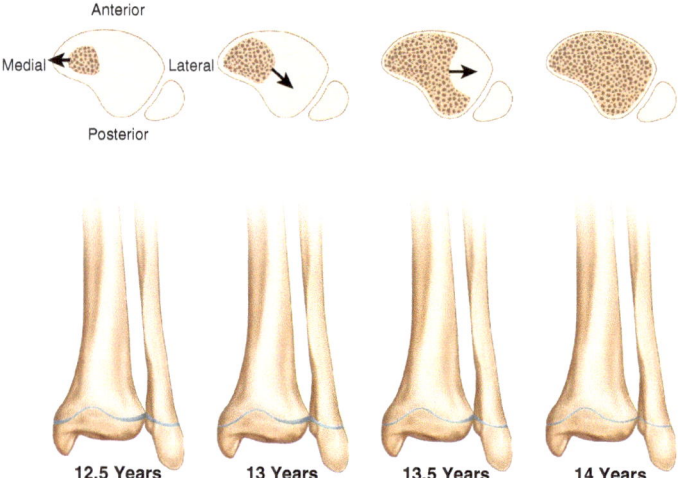

FIGURE 8.2 Distal tibia physis anatomy

8.6   Diagnosis

The child will typically present with a history of trauma such as a fall or twisting injury. The mechanism of injury dictates the amount of energy transferred to the tibia and will determine the extent of the bony injury as well as the soft tissue damage. Take note of the child's age and mobility status. Document whether the child is able to sit independently, crawl, bottom shuffle, cruise or is able to walk. Where the injury sustained is incongruent with history from the parents, non-accidental injury should be considered. Enquire about previous admissions to hospital and carefully document the clinical findings. It is important to liaise with the paediatric team in such cases.

The child will present with a limp, or a complete inability to weight bear on the affected side. Intra-articular injuries may present with a red, hot swollen joint, representing a haemarthrosis caused by ligamentous or bony injury.

8.7   When Examining the Tibia

- Inspect for lacerations, haematomas and ecchymosis.
- Examine for tenderness, and crepitus.
- Examine the knee and ankle joint for effusions, and ligamentous stability.
- Perform a complete distal neurological examination.
- Assess perfusion of the limb – capillary refill time, dorsalis pedis and posterior tibial pulses.
- Look for signs of compartment syndrome.

> - Non-accidental injury – perform a systematic examination looking for other long bone fractures, ecchymosis and retinal haemorrhages. Use a multidisciplinary approach to the patient with early involvement of the paediatricians, senior nursing staff and social services.
>
> - Compartment syndrome should be suspected in the presence of pain refractory to opiate analgesia, swelling, pain on passive flexion. Paraesthesia and pulselessness are late signs.

8.8   Imaging

- Anteroposterior and lateral radiographs of the tibia are usually adequate.
- Obtain views of the ankle and knee joints.
- Assess for comminution, displacement, translation, shortening and angulation.
- Computed tomography (CT) should be reserved for complex intra-articular injuries only, as there is a significant radiation dose delivered to the child.
- Magnetic resonance imaging (MRI) is used to assess ligamentous and meniscal pathology which are often associated with intra-articular fractures.

8.9   Proximal Tibial Fractures

Injuries affecting the proximal tibia include eminence (avulsion) injuries and tubercle fractures. These are considered in chapter (REFER TO KNEE CHAPTER).

8.9.1   Proximal Metaphysis Fracture (Cozen's Fracture)

Proximal tibial metaphyseal fractures are caused by a force applied to the lateral aspect of an extended knee, which causes the medial tibial physis to fail in tension. The fibula generally remains intact although it may undergo plastic deformation. The peak incidence of this injury is between 3 and 6 years when the femoral-tibial angle is growing towards valgus. Cozen described the development of a late tibial valgus deformity at around 12–24 months post injury. The aetiology of the deformity in uncertain however several theories have been described:

- Mechanical – avulsion of pes anserinus causing loss of medial tethering with intact fibula tethering, interposition of soft tissues within medial fracture gap increasing medial physeal growth, and expanding medial callus formation.

FIGURE 8.3 Cozen's fracture

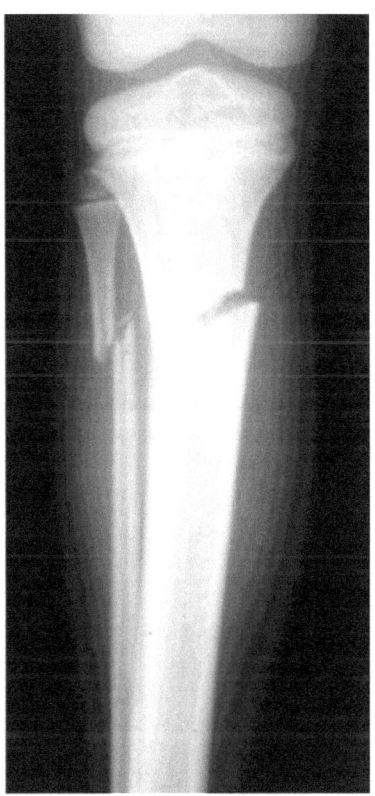

- Vascular – increase in blood flow to the medial tibial physis causes increased medial growth (Fig. 8.3).

There is no classification system for proximal tibial metaphyseal fractures. They are generally divided into complete or incomplete, displaced or undisplaced.

8.9.1.1 Treatment and Indications for Surgery

- Non-operative.
  Above knee cast – knee in 5–10° of flexion with varus moulding. Displaced fractures require closed reduction under anaesthesia and application of a varus moulded cast. Immobilise for 6 weeks, but the patient can weight bear

after 3 weeks. Wedging of the cast can be used to increase varus force.

• Operative.
  Interposed soft tissues (pes anserinus, periosteum) within the fracture site can prevent closed reduction. Removal of the soft tissues allows reduction and internal fixation is often not necessary.

8.9.1.2 Complications

• Valgus deformity – in the majority of cases spontaneously resolves over 18–36 months. Surgical intervention may be required in cases where there is persistent mechanical axis deviation of greater than 10° and no evidence of remodelling 18 months post injury. In the skeletally immature patient, medial hemiepiphysiodesis normally achieves correction within 1 year. However there is a 25% rate of mild rebound valgus deformity after removal of metalwork. In the skeletally mature patient, corrective osteotomies are indicated.
• Limb length discrepancy – asymmetrical growth can elongate the affected tibia.

8.10   Diaphyseal Tibial Fractures

Fractures of the tibial diaphysis and fibula are the third most common paediatric long bone injury, after forearm and femoral fractures. The fibula is fractured in 30% of tibial fractures. They are most commonly seen in children aged 11 years or below. Most fractures are due to a torsional force causing a spiral configuration at the middle/distal third of the tibia. Fractures of the diaphysis form a spectrum of patterns from low energy toddler's fractures to high-energy open fractures. The child will present with pain and a reluctance to weight bear on the affected side. On examination, there is local fracture site tenderness with exacerbation of pain when dorsiflexing the ankle. Examine for signs of compartment

TABLE 8.1 Suggested threshold for non-operative to operative management for diaphyseal tibial fractures in children

	<8 years	>8 years
Valgus	5°	5°
Varus	10°	5°
Shortening	10 mm	5 mm
Rotation	5°	5°
Angulation (apex anterior)	10°	5°
Angulation (apex posterior)	0°	0°

syndrome. Antero-posterior and lateral X-rays of the tibia and fibula including the knee and ankle joint are required.

8.10.1   AO Classification – Tibial Diaphysis

- Simple (A) – A1 Spiral, A2 Oblique (>30°), A3 Transverse.
- Wedge (B) – B1 Spiral wedge, B2 Bending wedge, B3 Fragmented wedge.
- Complex (C) – C1 Spiral, C2 Segmental, C3 Irregular.

8.10.2   Treatment and Indications for Surgery

- Non-operative.
  Closed reduction and above knee casting for 4–6 weeks.
  Indicated in toddlers fractures and displaced fractures with acceptable reduction, depending on age and remodelling potential (see Table 8.1 below).

- Operative.
  Indicated if there is unacceptable reduction outside the parameters described above. Furthermore, in cases of polytrauma to fascilitate mobilisation, or in the presence of compartment syndrome, neurovascular compromise or an open fracture. Treatment options include the use of K-wires, flexible intramedullary nails (Fig. 8.4) and plate fixation.

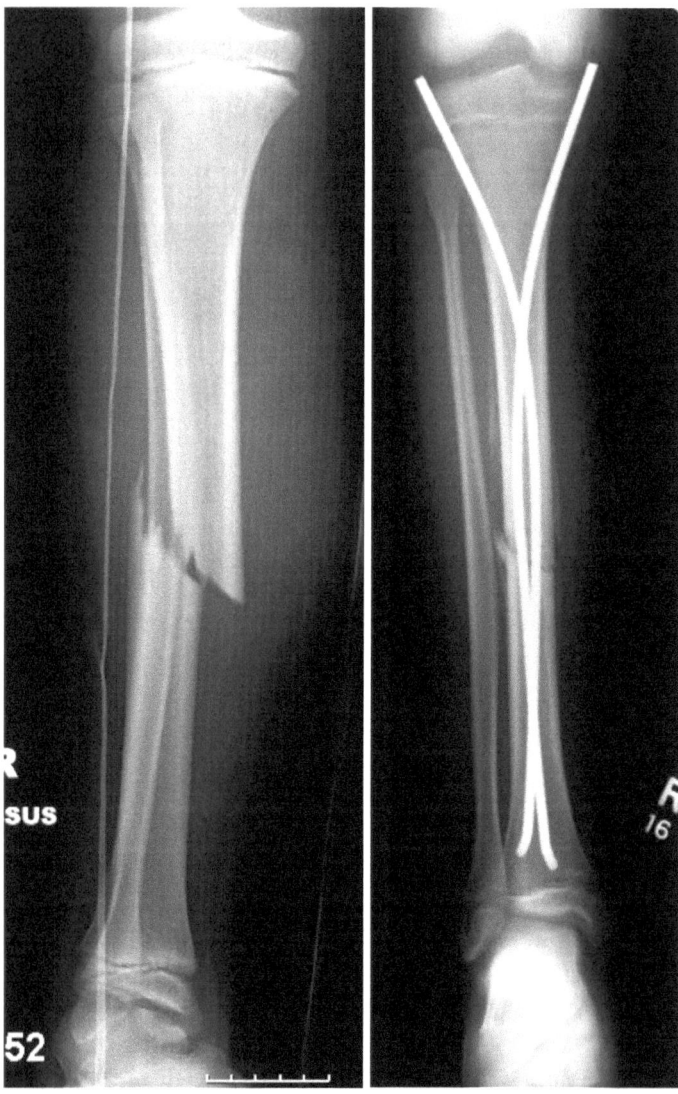

FIGURE 8.4 Pre- and postoperative radiographs of a tibial fracture treated with intra-medullary nailing

8.10.3   Complications

- Valgus malalignment – the anterolateral compartments of the leg will cause valgus deformity when associated with a fibula fracture.
- Varus malalignment – the anterior compartment of the leg will cause varus deformity when associated with an intact fibula due to its tethering effect.
- Compartment syndrome.
- Delayed union.

8.11   Toddler's Fractures (Childhood Accidental Spiral Tibial CAST Fractures)

Toddler's fractures are caused by external rotation of the foot with the knee in a fixed position producing a spiral fracture of the tibia. They tend to occur following a trivial twisting mechanism. They are most frequently seen in boys aged less than 6 years. It is an important differential to consider in the limping child. An internally rotated oblique view can be useful in identifying undisplaced fractures. Often the fracture is only visible on clinic review as the periosteal new bone forms at 7–14 days post injury. Occasionally bone scans may be required to identify fractures. The tibia will demonstrate diffuse increased uptake throughout the tibia (black tibia).

8.11.1   Treatment and Indications for Surgery

- Non-operative.
  Immobilisation in an above knee cast for 3–4 weeks.

- Operative.
  Manipulation under anaesthetic for displaced fractures and then immobilisation in an above knee cast for 3–4 weeks.

8.12   Open Fractures

Open fractures of the tibial diaphysis are normally the result of high energy trauma. Soft tissue injuries are typically less severe than in adults due to several important differences between adult and paediatric skeletons. The periosteum is often intact on the fracture concavity and can reform even after segmental bone loss. Devilatised, loose bone fragments should be removed as part of the debridement process.

Initial management should follow Advanced Trauma Life Support (ATLS) principles to identify life threatening injuries.

8.12.1   Gustillo-Anderson Classification

- Type 1 – wound <1 cm, low energy, "in/out injury".
- Type 2 – wound 1–10 cm, moderate energy, moderate soft tissue injury.
- Type 3.
    A – wound >10 cm, high energy, severely comminuted, segmental fractures, adequate soft tissue coverage.
    B – wound >10 cm, high energy, inadequate soft tissue, flap coverage required.
    C – wound >10 cm, high energy, neurovascular injury requiring repair/limb salvage.

8.12.2   Treatment and Indications for Surgery

- The treatment of open paediatric tibial fractures should follow the British Orthopaedic Association Standards for Trauma (BOAST 4) guidelines, which are evidence based and were developed by orthopaedic and plastic surgical bodies.
- Intravenous antibiotics within 3 h of injury.

- Tetanus prophylaxis (if not covered by school vaccinations).
- Neurovascular examination at regular intervals, especially after application of splints or casts.
- Vascular compromise requires immediate surgery with a maximum of 6 h of warm ischaemia time.
- Compartment syndrome – 4 compartment decompression, via a double incision approach.
- Wound handling only to remove gross contamination, and to allow photography.
- Wound cover with a saline soaked gauze and an impermeable film to prevent desiccation.
- Debridement of the soft tissues and bone is ideally performed by senior plastic and orthopaedic surgeons on a scheduled trauma list during normal working hours, unless there is marine, agricultural or sewage contamination.
- Definitive skeletal stabilisation and wound coverage ideally within 72 h, maximum 7 days.

8.12.3   Operative

Surgical options include the following:

- External fixation – unilateral frames are easy to apply and allow corrections in length and angulation.
- Flexible intramedullary nailing.
- Locked intramedullary nailing – older adolescents with closed physis.
- Internal fixation with plate.

8.12.4   Complications

- Non-union – <2% of cases.
- Delayed union – particularly in flexible titanium intramedullary nailing.

8.13   Distal Metaphyseal Fractures

Distal metaphyseal fractures are often greenstick injuries resulting in apex posterior angulation of the distal tibia. They are caused by a compressive force to the anterior tibial cortex and a tension force to the posterior tibial cortex, resulting in tearing of the overlying periosteum. This can result in a recurvatum deformity.

8.13.1   Treatment and Indications for Surgery

- Non-operative.
  Stable fractures can be treated with closed reduction and an above knee cast. Place the foot in plantar flexion to help reduce the fracture, and leave a cast on for 3-4 weeks. At this point, the cast can be changed to fascilitate a neutral ankle position.

- Operative.
  Unstable fractures can be treated with either closed reduction and percutaneous K-wire fixation or antegrade flexible nailing. Alternatively, open reduction and plate fixation can be used.

8.14   Synopsis

Paediatric tibial fractures represent some of the commonest fractures in trauma. The proximal and distal physis give rise to fractures which require specific management and can result in growth arrest and limb length discrepancy. High energy diaphyseal fractures can lead to compartment syndrome and should be promptly identified and treated. Multiple fractures or fractures in a non-ambulatory child should raise suspicion of non-accidental injury.

Key References

Setter KJ, Palomino KE. Pediatric tibia fractures: current concepts. Curr Opin Pediatr. 2006;18(1):30–5.

Mashru RP, Herman MJ, Pizzutillo PD. Tibial shaft fractures in children and adolescents. J Am Acad Orthop Surg. 2005;13(5):345–52.

Kay RM, Matthys GA. Pediatric ankle fractures: evaluation and treatment. J Am Acad Orthop Surg. 2001;9(4):268–78.

Chapter 9
Ankle Injuries

Anna C. Peek and Claudia Maizen

9.1 Introduction

In a monograph in 1898, Poland described physeal fractures at the ankle and established the principle that in children, ligaments are stronger than physeal cartilage. This, combined with anatomy of the physis and direction in which it closes, gives rise to a pattern of injury particular to children and young adults.

The ankle mortise is bound by three ligamentous structures: the tibiofibular syndesmotic ligaments, the deltoid ligament medially, and laterally the anterior, posterior talofibular ligaments and calcaneofibular ligaments (Fig. 9.1). Because of their relative strength, they rarely fail, but instead physeal elements are avulsed by them. The tibiofibular syndesmosis consists of four ligaments, the anterior and posterior inferior tibiofibular ligaments, the transverse tibiofibular ligament, and the interosseous tibiofibular ligament. The interosseous

A. C. Peek, FRCS (Tr & Orth) (✉)
T&O SpR Percivall Pott Rotation, London, UK
e-mail: annapeek@doctors.org.uk

C. Maizen, MD, FRCS (Orth)
Consultant Orthopaedic and Trauma Surgeon,
The Royal London and Barts and The London Children's
Hospitals, Barts Health, London, UK

N.A. Aresti et al. (eds.), *Paediatric Orthopaedic Trauma in Clinical Practice*, In Clinical Practice,
DOI 10.1007/978-1-4471-6756-3_9,
© Springer-Verlag London Ltd. 2015

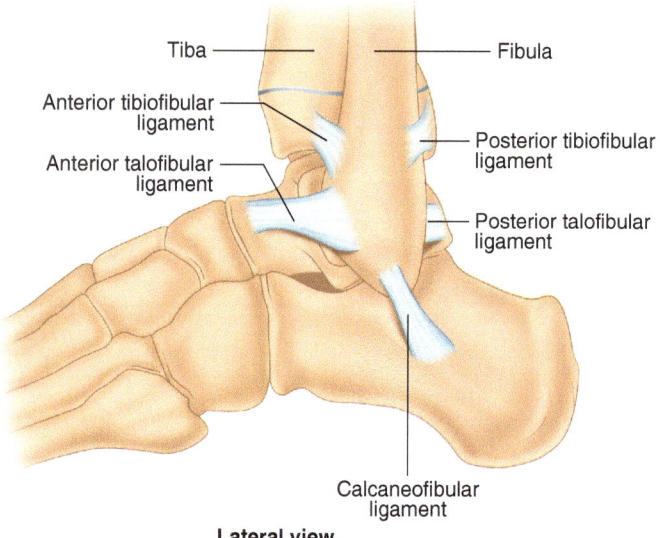

Lateral view

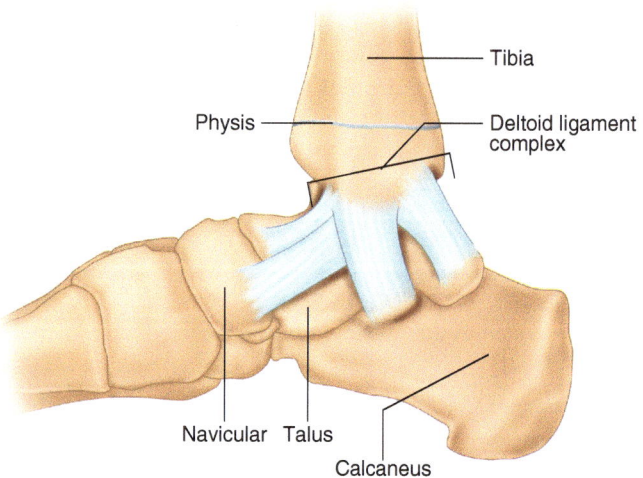

Medial view

FIGURE 9.1 Diagram showing the ligaments around the ankle

tibiofibular ligament is strongest and primary stabiliser of the syndesmosis.

The distal tibial ossification centre appears between 6 and 24 months of age and the distal fibular ossific centre around 9–24 months of age. The medial malleolus ossifies around 7 years old. The pattern of closure of the distal tibial physis is important:

1. The centre closes first (this region is known as Kump's bump or Poland's hump);
2. Followed by the medial and;
3. Finally the lateral side.

This is important in transitional fracture patterns. The process takes around 18 months and is usually complete around the age of 15 years in girls, 2 years later in boys (Fig. 9.2).

9.2 Incidence

- Common injuries, accounting for 28–35% of all physeal fractures.
- More common in boys than girls.
- 58% of injuries occur during sports.
- Bimodal distribution with small peak in pre-school children and larger peak in adolescents.

9.3 Classification

Distal tibial physeal fractures can be classified anatomically or according to their mechanism of injury.

9.3.1 Anatomical

The Salter-Harris classification can be used as with other physeal fractures. Its advantages are its simplicity and widespread use. It does not, however, describe the forces involved in the injury or differentiate between shearing and crushing

FIGURE 9.2 Diagram showing
the pattern of fusion of the
distal tibial physis

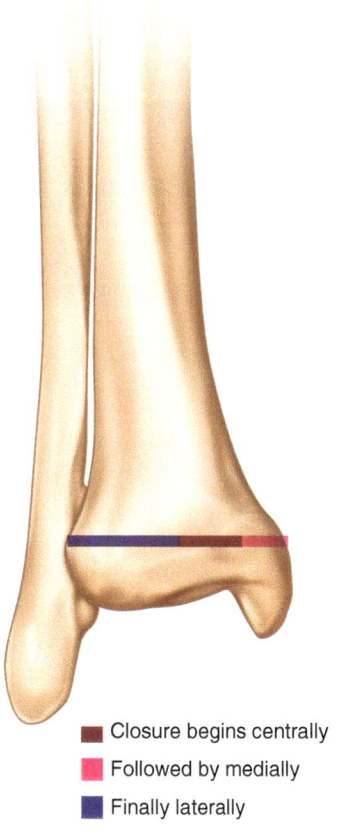

■ Closure begins centrally
■ Followed by medially
■ Finally laterally

mechanisms which carry different prognoses with regards to
later growth disturbance.

9.3.2   Mechanism of Injury

The Dias-Tachdjian is the most widely accepted classification
based on mechanism of injury and deforming force. Described in
1978, additional categories including axial compression fractures

and transitional fractures were added in 1985. It is a modification of the Lauge-Hansen classification. As with the Lauge-Hansen, the first word relates to the position of the foot at the time of injury and second word the deforming force (Fig. 9.3).

- Supination-External rotation:
  - This is the most common mechanism encountered.
  - Grade 1: Salter-Harris type 2 fracture of the distal tibia; the fracture line extends in a spiral proximally and medially, the distal fragment is displaced posteriorly.
  - Grade 2: with further external rotation there is an antero-inferior to posterosuperior spiral fracture of the fibula.

- Supination-Inversion (Adduction):
  - Grade 1: distal fibular avulsion (either Salter-Harris type 1 or 2).
  - Grade 2: further inversion causes a tibial fracture, most commonly a Salter-Harris type 3 or 4. The injury passes through the medial malleolus.

- Supination-Plantarflexion.
  - The tibial epiphysis is forced posteriorly, usually a Salter-Harris type 1 or 2. The fibula remains intact. The tibial fragment may be difficult to appreciate on an AP radiograph. Closed reduction may be difficult as the torn anterior periosteum or the anterior neurovascular bundle may cause soft tissue interposition.

- Pronation-Eversion (external rotation).
  - A Salter-Harris type 1 or 2 fracture of the distal tibia with a transverse fibula fracture. The distal fragments are displaced laterally. Alternatively there may be a Salter-Harris type 3 fracture through the medial malleolus, exiting medial to the midline. This is one of the rare injuries that may be associated with diastasis of the ankle joint in children.

- Axial compression.
  - This causes a Salter-Harris type 5 fracture. Initial radiographs show no abnormality, but follow-up demonstrates growth arrest.

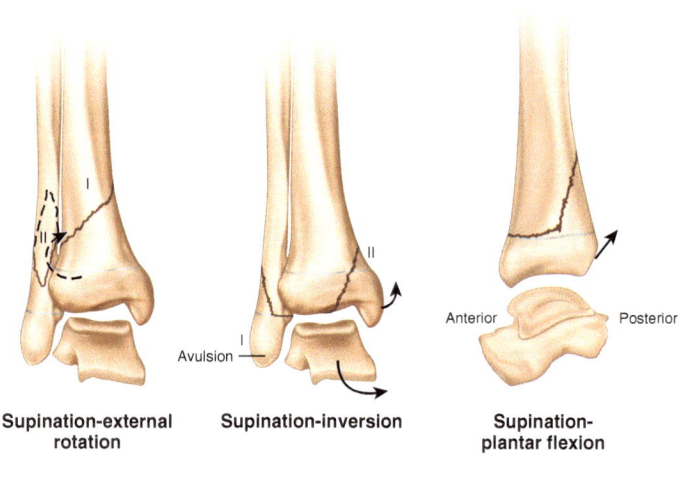

Supination-external rotation

Supination-inversion

Supination-plantar flexion

Anterior   Posterior

Avulsion

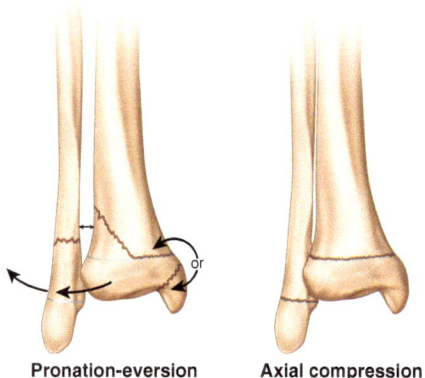

Pronation-eversion

Axial compression

FIGURE 9.3 (**a–d**) Summary of the Dias-Tachdjian classification

9.3.3   Transitional Fractures

These fractures occur in the adolescent with a partially closed distal tibial physis.

- Tillaux fractures (see Fig. 9.4).

  - Described by Paul Jules Tillaux, a Parisian surgeon (1834–1904).
  - External rotation injury causes avulsion of the antero-lateral distal tibial epiphysis, at the attachment of the anterior inferior tibiofibular ligament.
  - The injury only occurs when the central and medial parts of the tibial physis have closed but the lateral part remains open.
  - The typical age is between 13 and 16 years.
  - The injury is commonly missed.

- Triplane fractures.

  - Described by Lynn in 1972, these occur in the axial, sagittal, and coronal planes.
  - These are also external rotation injuries, but tend to occur in a slightly younger age group than Tillaux fractures (10–16 years old).

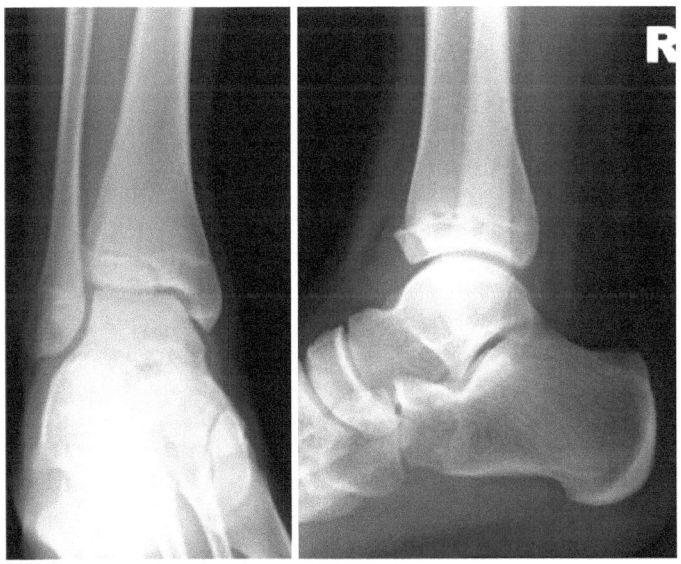

FIGURE 9.4 AP and lateral radiographs demonstrating a Tillaux fracture

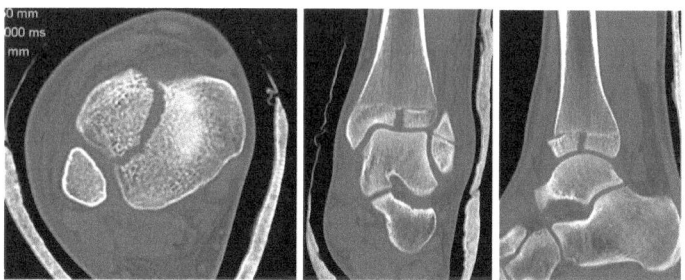

FIGURE 9.5 CT scan illustrating the typical anatomical location of the Tillaux fragment

- On the AP radiograph the fracture looks like a Salter-Harris type 3 fracture, but on the lateral radiograph the metaphyseal fragment is visible (Fig. 9.5).
- The epiphyseal fragment may be in 2 or even 3 parts. Rarely, the fracture line through the epiphysis exits extra-articular through the medial malleolus.
- In 50% of cases the fibula is fractured.
- CT is very helpful in evaluation of the fracture and the degree of articular displacement (Figs. 9.6 and 9.7).

9.3.4   Lawnmower Injuries

Lawnmowers and high energy road traffic accidents are the most common causes of severe open ankle fractures and are treated along the same principles as any open fracture, with early antibiotics, copious washout and debridement, skeletal stabilisation and soft tissue cover. External fixation may be used but the physis should be avoided in placing the pins. Soft tissue cover may be obtained through local, free or even cross extremity flaps.

Where there is disruption of the tendo Achilles in these injuries, reconstruction of the tendon is not always required as dense posterior scarring may produce a physiological result, or a secondary late reconstruction may be undertaken.

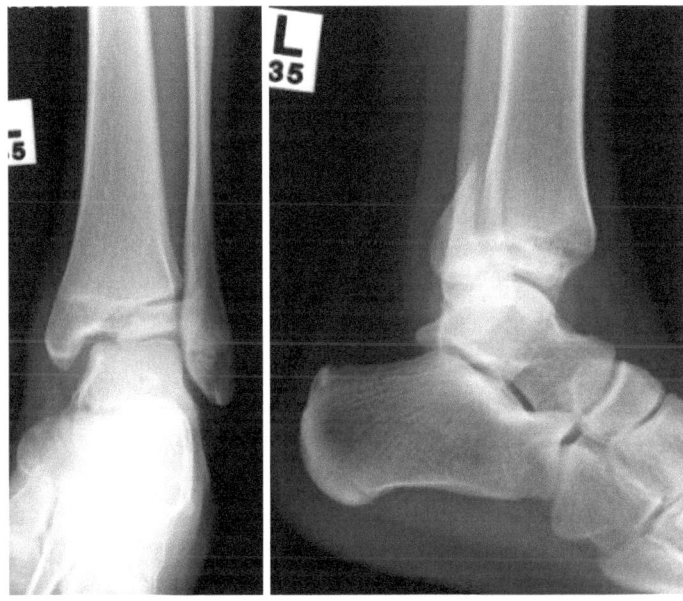

FIGURE 9.6 Triplane fracture radiographs. Notice how the fracture looks like a Salter-Harris type 3 on the AP radiograph and a Salter-Harris type 2 on the lateral radiograph

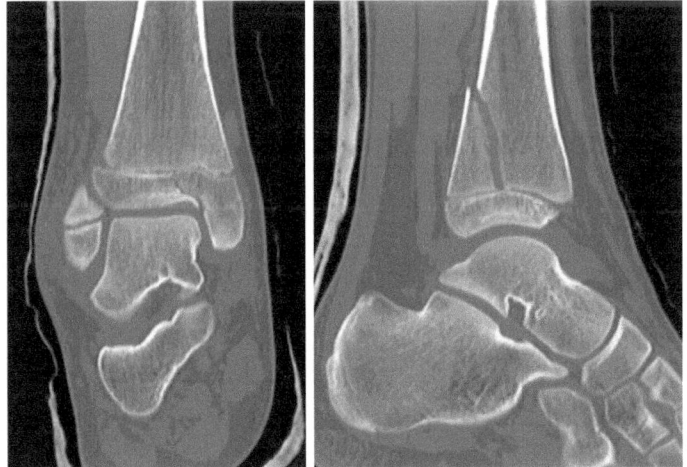

FIGURE 9.7 Triplane fracture. The sagittal and coronal elements of the fracture are well demonstrated on CT scanning

9.4   Treatment

The majority of fractures can be treated by closed reduction and immobilisation. When a fracture requires reduction, consideration should be given to the age and degree of co-operation of the child: it is often preferable for the child to have a general anaesthesia as repeated or forceful attempts at reduction may damage the physis. Reduction is more likely to be successful and atraumatic to the physis if the child is relaxed.

The Dias-Tachdjian classification will help guide the method of reduction, which should reverse the injuring force, for example in supination–external rotation injuries the foot should be placed in pronation and internal rotation.

Acceptable degrees of residual angulation for children with 2 or more years of growth remaining have been suggested as 15° of apex anterior angulation, 10° of valgus, no varus.

In the case of Tillaux and triplane fractures, there is evidence that residual displacement was significantly less in patients in whom a pre-operative CT scan was carried out.

Fractures which remain displaced >2 mm require open reduction and fixation. The approach can be anteromedial or anterolateral depending on the fracture configuration. Any intervening periosteum must be removed. For triplane fractures the metaphyseal fragment is usually best reduced first followed by the epiphyseal fragment. Arthroscopically assisted paercutaneous fixation of triplane fractures has been described.

Fixation is usually achieved with epiphyseal and metaphyseal screws where appropriate. In children the physis should be avoided, but in adolescents with transitional fracture patterns this is not a concern.

The need for subsequent removal of metalware remains controversial. A recent metanalysis found no evidence to either support or refute removal of metalware.

9.5   Complications and Follow-Up

9.5.1   Growth Disturbance

Premature physeal closure (Fig. 9.8), either symmetrical or asymmetrical, is rare but well described. A series of 137 Salter-Harris 1 and 2 injuries reported an overall rate of 39%, with a rate of 54% in patients having sustained Lauge-Hansen pronation-abduction type injuries. A previous smaller

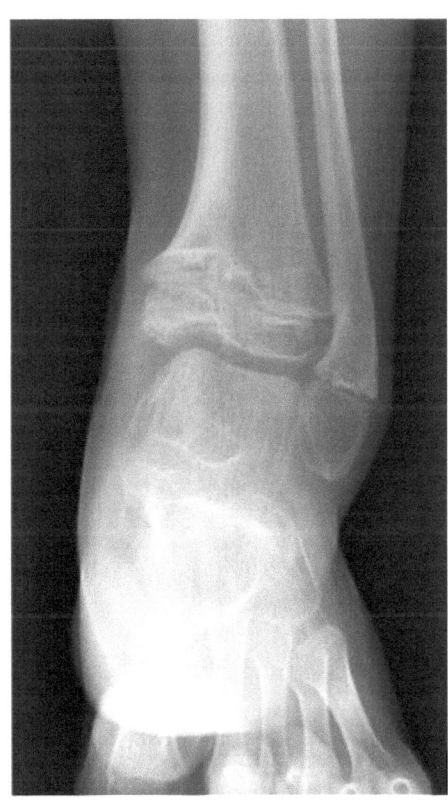

FIGURE 9.8 AP radiograph of growth arrest in an ankle

series found a similar rate in Salter-Harris 3 and 4 injuries. Post reduction displacement was the strongest predictor for premature physeal arrest. A residual gap in the physis (>3 mm) may represent periosteal entrapment and, if present, the risk of premature growth arrest increases to 60%.

On plain radiographs an osseous bar may be visible. Harris growth arrest lines are helpful in asymmetrical growth arrest where they will be divergent from the line of the physis or absent. Harris growth lines usually appear 6–12 weeks after injury. A continuous line parallel to the physis without focal defects is reassuring.

Patients should be followed up until skeletal maturity or until a Harris growth arrest line parallel to the physis can be demonstrated.

In the normal ankle the distal fibular metaphysis moves distally in relation to the tibial metaphysis, due to more rapid growth proximally and ligamentous traction. This can compensate partially for an isolated fibular growth arrest. If there is isolated distal tibial growth arrest the ongoing fibula growth may move the shaft and proximal portion of the fibula more proximally; however a varus deformity may also develop.

If there are signs of growth arrest any metalware in situ should be removed. Treatment thereafter depends on the remaining growth potential but may include resection of the physeal bar, epiphysiodesis to prevent a varus/valgus deformity, or indeed a wedge osteotomy, should such a deformity be present.

9.5.2   Malunion

Varus or valgus malunion may occur either secondary to partial growth arrest (5%) or due to a primary malunion (4.5%). Residual displacement occurs significantly less in patients in whom a pre-operative CT scan was carried out.

Studies have shown around a 60% rate of external rotation (compared to the uninjured side) following Salter-Harris 1 and 2 distal tibial fractures. Many of these patients also have associated physeal widening. Functional deficit rarely results, but some patients and their families notice the difference between the limbs.

Any residual articular displacement in the weight bearing area may cause early degenerative change. Following triplane fractures, early good results at an average of 24 months deteriorates when patients are seen an average 6 years post injury, in those patients where >2 mm of displacement remains post reduction. However this is not the case in patients where the fracture line exited extra-articular through the medial malleolus.

9.6   Talar Dome Osteochondral Lesions

9.6.1   Background

Fractures of the chondral surface of the talus are more common in adolesence compared with talar fractures proper. Lesions to the lateral surface are most common and more symptomatic. They are thought to be as a result of the anterolateral aspect of the talus abutting on the medial flbula in the extremeties of dorsiflexion and inversion. Conversely, the medial surface is damaged in plantarflexion and inversion. Patients often present with symptoms complaining of a sprain, with persistent pain and swelling.

9.6.2   Classification

The Berndt and Hardy classification is perhaps the most comprehensive for osteochondral talus injuries and has formed the basis of other modified classification systems. It is based on an ankle mortise view.

Stage 1 – subchondral fracture
Stage 2 – partially detached fragment
Stage 3 – detached fragment which remains undisplaced
Stage 4 – displaced and detached fragment.

Plain radiographs may miss up to 50% of lesions, therefore MRI/CT or repeat radiographs after 2–4 weeks are indicated where there is a clinical suspicion. The Bristol and Andersson classifications are based on MRI and take into account the presence of bone cysts and oedema surrounding the lesion, which have prognositic significance.

9.6.3   Treatment

It is important to first distinguish bettween acute and chronic lesions as they require different treatments. In acute injuries, stage 1 and 2 lesions can be treated non operatively with immobilisation for around 6 weeks, followed by physiotherapy. Patients with stage 3 or 4 lesions benefit from surgery, which is mainly arthroscopic. Options include microfracture or drilling the lesion, fixation with absorbable screws or bone grafting and fixation.

9.7   Ankle Ligament Injuries

Ankle sprains/ligament injuries are commonly seen. They are brought about by rotational injuries, affecting the lateral ligament complexes, and may be associated with medial ligament injuries or fractures. They present with swelling and tenderness around the medial maleolus or tip of the fibula. They may be associated with instabilty. Below the age of 10–12, around 80% of injuries are associated with a periosteal, chondral or osseous avulsion (most commonly from the tip of the fibula).

Following an acute presentation, patients are actively rehabilitated unless there is an avulsion injury visible on a radiograph, in which case a short period of immobilisation in a below knee cast would be indicated. Around 10% of patients may have ongoing symptoms of instability. In these patients, ligament reconstruction may well be indicated.

Key References

Rockwood CA, Wilkins KE, Beaty JH, Kasser JR, editors. Rockwood and Wilkins' fractures in children. 6th ed. Philadelphia: Lippincott Williams & Wilkins; 2006.

Herring JA, Tachdjian MO, Texas Scottish Rite Hospital for Children, editors. Tachdjian's pediatric orthopaedics. 4th ed. Philadelphia: Saunders/Elsevier; 2008. 3 p.

Seel EH, Noble S, Clarke NMP, Uglow MG. Outcome of distal tibial physeal injuries. J Pediatr Orthop B. 2011;20(4):242–8.

Ertl JP, Barrack RL, Alexander AH, VanBuecken K. Triplane fracture of the distal tibial epiphysis. Long-term follow-up. J Bone Joint Surg Am. 1988;70(7):967–76.

Cutler L, Molloy A, Dhukuram V, Bass A. Do CT scans aid assessment of distal tibial physeal fractures? J Bone Joint Surg Br. 2004;86(2):239–43.

Phan VC, Wroten E, Yngve DA. Foot progression angle after distal tibial physeal fractures. J Pediatr Orthop. 2002;22(1):31–5.

Hynes D, O'Brien T. Growth disturbance lines after injury of the distal tibial physis. Their significance in prognosis. J Bone Joint Surg Br. 1988;70(2):231–3.

Vosburgh CL, Gruel CR, Herndon WA, Sullivan JA. Lawn mower injuries of the pediatric foot and ankle: observations on prevention and management. J Pediatr Orthop. 1995;15(4):504–9.

Chapter 10
Fractures of the Foot

Keng Suan Khor and Nima Heidari

10.1   Epidemiology

Fractures of the foot are uncommon in childhood and account for 5–8% of all fractures and 7% of all physeal injuries. The forefoot is the most common site of injury comprising two-thirds of the fractures.

The high percentage of radiolucent skeletal structures and the resilient soft tissue coverage contribute to the difficulty in evaluating the severity of injury and compartment syndrome of the foot may occur in the absence of any fractures. Fall from a height is the most common mechanism of injury in forefoot fractures, whereas fractures of the mid- and hind-foot are associated with high-energy trauma.

———

K.S. Khor, MBBS, BSc (Hons), MRCS (✉)
T&O SpR Percivall Pott Rotation, London, UK
e-mail: kengsuan@gmail.com

N. Heidari, MBBS, MSc, FRCS (Tr&Orth)
Consultant Orthopaedic and Trauma Surgeon,
The Royal London Limb Reconstruction Service,
The Royal London and Barts and The London
Children's Hospitals, Barts Health, London, UK

N.A. Aresti et al. (eds.), *Paediatric Orthopaedic Trauma in Clinical Practice*, In Clinical Practice,
DOI 10.1007/978-1-4471-6756-3_10,
© Springer-Verlag London Ltd. 2015

10.2   Diagnosis

10.2.1   Clinical Features

A full assessment of the injured foot includes a history and clinical examination. The injury is often not witnessed in the child. A careful examination of the soft tissues and observation to assess the child's ability to bear weight on the injured limb is essential.

Crush injuries carry the risk of compartment syndrome even in the absence of fractures. Close monitoring of a significantly swollen foot is mandatory and the patient should be admitted for elevation. Pressure recording maybe helpful in the unconscious polytraumatised patient but otherwise the decision to perform compartment decompression should be based on clinical suspicion.

Open fractures require administration of tetanus vaccine, antibiotics, debridement and skeletal stabilisation in accordance with established protocols such as the BOAST 4 guidelines.

10.3   Imaging

Routine radiographs include AP and oblique views. When displacement or dislocation at the tarsometatarsal joints is suspected or a fracture of the talus or calcaneum may be present, a true lateral projection is mandatory. In fractures of the calcaneum, an axial projection provides information about calcaneal widening and deformity in the coronal plane.

A CT scan is invaluable in delineating the exact anatomy of calcaneal fractures and aids in preoperative planning. An MRI scan is useful in the diagnosis and assessment of ligamentous injuries. These imaging modalities are also indicated when a tarsal coalition is suspected.

Accessory bones can be mistaken for fractures and are occasionally bipartite. If doubt exists as to whether they are fractured, then either a CT scan to visualize the bone more clearly or an MRI scan which will show bone oedema and soft tissue contusion in the presence of a fracture can help to make a diagnosis (Table 10.1).

10.4   Fractures of Calcaneum

10.4.1   Epidemiology

Calcaneal fractures account for 1–2% of all fractures in adults and some 65% are intra-articular. In contrast this is a rare injury in children (below the age of 14) with the majority (70%) being extra-articular. In adolescents as the skeleton nears maturity the fracture patterns tend to resemble those of the adult with a greater proportion (60–80%) being intra-articular.

As in the adult population the majority of injuries are as a result of a fall from a height (47%), road traffic accidents (15%) and lawnmowers (13%). Up to one-third are associated with other fractures, with lower extremity fractures occurring more frequently than lumbar spine fractures. Fractures in children and adolescents also tend to be less comminuted. This may reflect the fact that these fractures in children are much lower energy injuries and the more cartilaginous immature calcaneum predisposes it to simpler fracture patterns.

10.4.2   Classification

One of the early and most widely accepted classifications of calcancal fractures was proposed by Essex-Lopresti. This was then modified by Schmidt and Weiner for use in the paediatric population (Table 10.2).

10.4.3   Diagnosis

Children sustaining fractures of the calcaneum are likely to have been involved in high-energy trauma. With displaced fractures, the injury to the soft tissue envelope will be directly

TABLE 10.1 Accessory and sesamoid bones of the foot and ankle (Mellado et al. 2003)

Accessory bone	Prevalence (%)	Clinical significance	Differential diagnosis
Os trigonum	1–25	Synchondrotic degeneration or tear Posterior ankle impingement syndrome Flexor hallucis longus tendon entrapment	Shepherd's fracture Cedell's fracture Pseudoarthrosis
Accessory navicular	2–12	Synchondrotic degeneration or tear Posterior tibial tendon dysfunction or tear	Navicular tuberosity avulsion fracture
Os sustentaculi	0.3–0.4	Synchondrotic degeneration Painful syndrome	Isolated fracture of the sustentaculum tali
Os intermetatarseum	1.2–10	Painful syndrome	Lisfranc fracture dislocation
Os supranaviculare	1	Painful syndrome	Cortical avulsion fracture of the navicular or talar head
Os vesalianum	0.1	Painful syndrome	Avulsion fracture at the base of the fifth metatarsal
Os calcaneus secundarius	0.6–7	None	Avulsion fracture of the anterosuperior calcaneal process
Os subtibiale	0.9	None	Medial malleollus avulsion fracture
Os subfibulare	2.1	Painful syndrome	Lateral malleolus avulsion fracture
Os peroneum	9	Painful os peroneum syndrome	Bipartite os peroneum Painful os vesalianum
Hallux sesamoid bones	Close to 100	Fracture, stress fracture, diastasis	Bipartite sesamoid

TABLE 10.2 Schmidt and Weiner classification of calcaneal fractures in children

Extra-articular	1	A. Tuberosity or apophysis B. Sustentaculum tali C. Anterior process D. Distal inferomedial aspect E. Small avulsions off body	
	2	A. Beak fracture B. Avulsion fracture of Achilles tendon insertion	
	3	Linear fracture not involving subtalar joint	
Intra-articular	4	Linear fracture involving subtalar joint	
	5	A. Tongue type	
		B. Joint depression type	
Tissue loss	6	Significant bone loss of posterior aspect with loss of Achilles tendon insertion	

related to the energy of the injury. The foot is often very swollen with substantial bruising and blistering. The possibility of compartment syndrome must be considered.

Standard radiographs for the calcaneum include the lateral and axial projections. Oblique views may help with identifying anterior process fractures. Bohler's angle has been used in determining the presence of an intra-articular fracture and to quantify the degree of displacement. In adults the angle is quoted as being between 20° and 40°. In young children, the range is higher than in the adult, due to the incomplete ossification of the calcaneus. It then rapidly increases with age. By the age of 7 years the estimated mean angle is 42°. The angle tends to decline towards adult values as the child enters adolescence. Measuring the non-injured foot angle is recommended for comparative purposes, although in the case of displaced fractures the modality of choice is a CT scan.

10.4.4   Treatment

The great majority of calcaneal fractures in growing young children can be treated non-operatively due to the potential for remodelling. In the adolescent, fractures resemble the patterns seen in adults and the remodelling potential is greatly reduced. In this group, excellent results have been reported with the operative treatment of displaced intra-articular fractures.

The difficulty in determining how to treat calcaneal fractures in children lies with deciding whether the remaining remodelling process will sufficiently correct the ensuing fracture deformity.

10.4.4.1 Non-operative Treatment

Once the threat of compartment syndrome has abated, a below knee plaster maybe applied for comfort. It should be left on for 6 weeks during which excessive bruising or blistering should be regularly reviewed, potentially with windows in the plaster.

10.4.4.2 Operative Treatment

The extended lateral approach is typically the approach used for open reduction, internal fixation. Surgery should be performed once the soft tissue swelling has settled. A delay of up to 2 weeks is acceptable. A suction drain is advocated for the first 24 h to avoid a wound haematoma that can lead to wound breakdown. Following the closure of the wound, a below knee back slab is applied and the limb elevated. There is a high rate of wound complication and so the wound should be reviewed after 24 h. Protection of the limb in a plaster is advisable for 6 weeks. The wound should be reviewed regularly. During this period the patient should not bear weight through the foot (Fig. 10.1).

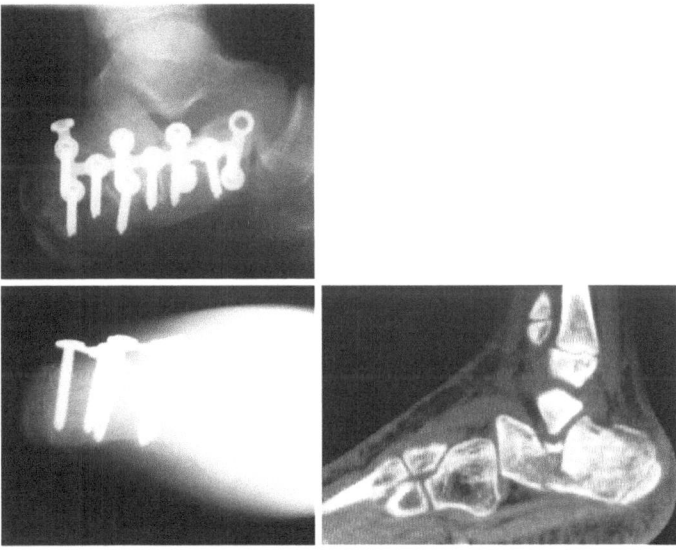

FIGURE 10.1 Comminuted fracture of a calcaneum in a 13 year old child – a CT scan of the injury and post operative radiographs (Reprinted with permission from Benson et al. (2009) *Children's Orthopaedics and Fractures*, Springer)

10.4.5   Delayed Presentation

Many undisplaced and low energy calcaneal fractures are missed in younger children. These tend to heal without consequence. In children below the age of 10, there is good evidence that even articular displacement remodels and the final outcome is good.

10.5   Fractures of Talus

10.5.1   Epidemiology

Fractures of the talus are rare and account for only 0.008% of all childhood fractures. These are often high-energy injuries and concomitant injuries must be ruled out. Significant consequences of these fractures include avascular necrosis as well as post-traumatic arthritis due to malalignment.

10.5.2   Types of Fractures

Fractures most commonly occur at the talar neck, which were classified by Hawkins (Table 10.3). This classifies the injury according to the degree of displacement of the talar neck and subluxation of the tibio-talar, subtalar and talo-navicular joints. The Marti/Weber classification is also commonly used (Table 10.4). Eberl reported less severe injuries (Marti/Weber type I and II) in younger children, in contrast to older children who were prone to fracture-dislocations requiring operative fixation (Marti/Weber type III and IV). This may be due to the more flexible cartilaginous talus, which is less likely to fracture.

10.5.3   Treatment

Non-operative Treatment

The foot and ankle are immobilised in a cast for 6–8 weeks. The patient is not allowed to bear weight on the injured leg.

TABLE 10.3 Hawkins Classification of talar neck fractures

Type I	Undislocated talar neck fractures
Type II	Dislocation at the subtalar joint
Type III	Dislocation at the subtalar and ankle joints
Type IV	Dislocation at the subtalar, talonavicular and ankle joints

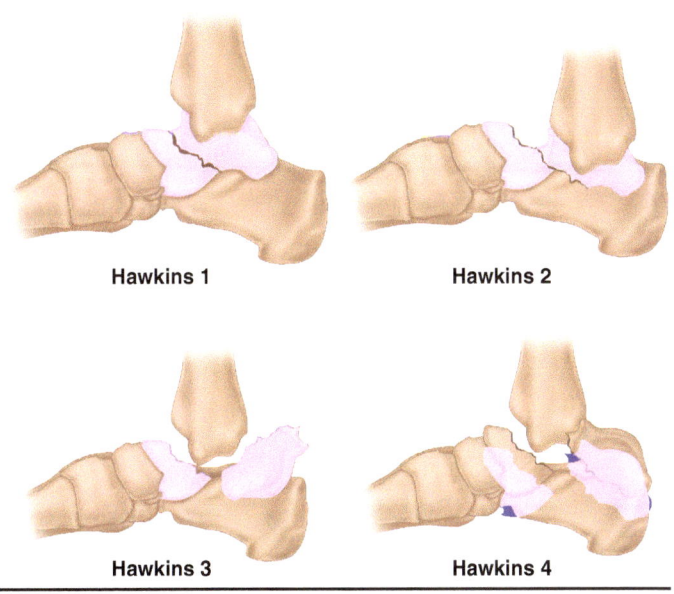

Reprinted with permission from Lasanianos et al. (2015) *Trauma and Orthopaedic Classifications: A Comprehensive Overview*, Springer

20° of plantar flexion at the ankle will help reduce any displacement of the talus. In undisplaced fractures, a below knee cast will suffice.

10.5.3.1 Operative Treatment

Open reduction and internal fixation to achieve anatomical reduction will reduce the risk of avascular necrosis in more severe or displaced fractures [Fig. 10.2].

TABLE 10.4 Marti/Weber classification of talar fractures

Type i	Distal talar neck and talar head fractures, peripheral fractures and osteochandral flakes
Type ii	Undisplaced talar neck and corpus fractures
Type iii	Dislocated talar neck and corpus fractures
Type iv	Proximal talar neck fractures with corpus tali luxated out of the intermalleolar space or comminuted fracture

Type I : Distal talar neck and talar head fractures, peripheral fractures and osteochandral flakes

Type II : Undisplaced talar neck and corpus fractures

Type III : Dislocated talar neck and corpus fractures

Type IV : Proximal talar neck fractures with corpus tali luxated out of the intermalleolar space or comminuted fracture

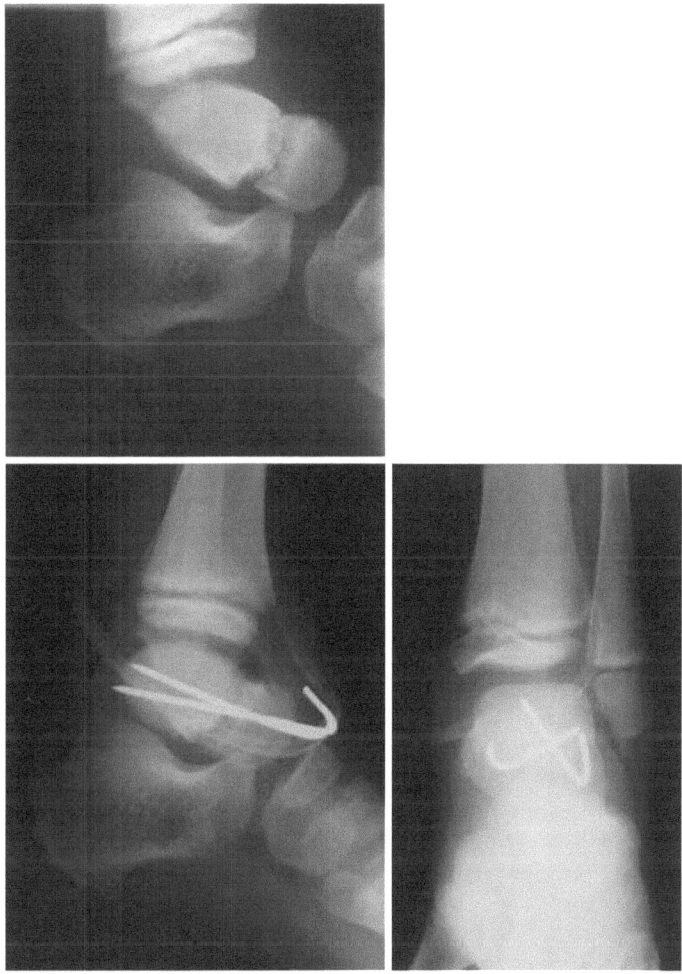

FIGURE 10.2 Talar neck fracture (Hawkin's type II). With fixation (Reprinted with permission from Benson et al. (2009) *Children's Orthopaedics and Fractures*, Springer)

10.5.3.2 Follow-Up

Regular radiographs should be taken to monitor for evidence of subchondral osteopenia of the talar dome, which is an indicator of talar viability. Hawkins described this subchondral lucency when there was a good vascular supply in the setting of disuse. A negative Hawkins sign is observed when there is progression to sclerosis, indicative of avascular necrosis (AVN). In suspected AVN, the patient should be non-weight bearing for a further 4 weeks and be investigated with an MRI scan. Once AVN is confirmed, walking aids may be needed for mobilisation and subsequent repeat MRI or bone scans may be needed for monitoring.

10.6   Midfoot Fractures

Midfoot injuries in children are rare and are often caused by high-energy trauma.

10.6.1   Chopart Joint Injuries

Chopart fracture-dislocations are rare, high-energy injuries, which involve the mid-tarsal joints. Inversion injuries result in medial dislocations whereas eversion injuries cause lateral dislocations. Urgent reduction is required as these injuries have a poor prognosis.

10.6.2   Fractures of the Navicular

The navicular serves as the keystone to the medial arch of the foot. Displaced fractures must be treated with open reduction and internal fixation to maintain the length and height of the medial arch. After surgery and for non-displaced fractures, patients are immobilised in a Sarmiento cast for 4–6 weeks. Once there is evidence of clinical and radiological union, they can increasingly bear more weight through the foot. Metalwork is removed 3–4 months postoperatively.

10.7   Metatarsal Fractures

10.7.1   Epidemiology

In children, up to two-thirds of all fractures of the foot involve the metatarsal bones. Fractures of the second, third, and fourth metatarsals are frequently associated with fractures of another metatarsal, whereas the majority of first and fifth metatarsal fractures are isolated and account for 85% of all metatarsal fractures. They occur as a result of direct or indirect forces. Fractures sustained at the base of the metatarsals tend to be due to indirect force, and shaft and head fractures result from direct trauma to the foot.

Children below the age of 5 tend to have more fractures of the first metatarsal whereas those over the age of 5 tend to have fractures of the fifth metatarsal. Fractures of the base of the fifth metatarsal are the most common isolated injury of the foot. The fracture line is often perpendicular to shaft of the bone and should not be confused with the proximal apophysis (os vesalanium), which is parallel to the long axis of the bone (Fig. 10.3).

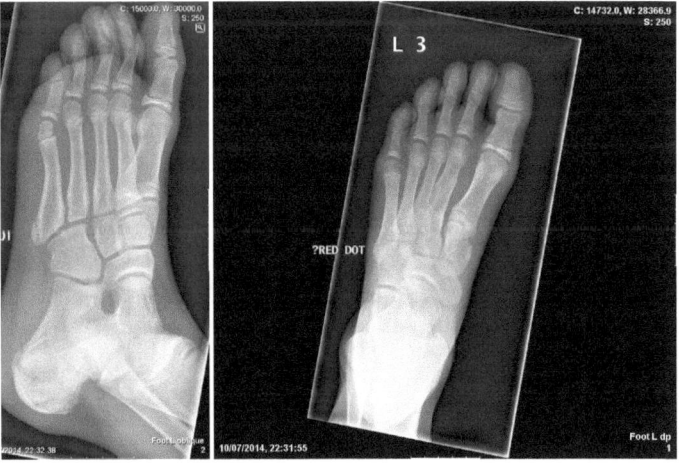

Figure 10.3 Base of fifth metatarsal fracture and apophysis – AP and oblique view of the same patient

10.7.2   Diagnosis

Fractures of the base of the metatarsals may indicate an accompanying injury to the tarsometatarsal joints. Multiple metatarsal fractures indicate a severe injury and the treating clinician must be cognizant of the possibility of compartment syndrome.

10.7.2.1 Stress Fractures

Although more commonly reported in the adult, these fractures are rarely observed in children. Stress fractures should be considered in the differential diagnosis of young athletes. If the fracture is not initially visible on initial radiographs, repeat radiographs 2–3 weeks later may show callus formation. Increasingly, MRI is recognized as the study of choice in these injuries. The treatment is generally non-operative with cast immobilisation for up to 6 weeks and the child can bear weight through the foot once the symptoms have settled.

10.7.3   Treatment , Indication for Surgery, Follow-Up

The majority of metatarsal fractures can be treated non-operatively. A backslab and elevation for the first few days will allow the swelling to reduce. A cast can then be applied for 3–6 weeks and the child allowed to mobilise as comfort allows in the cast. Grossly displaced fractures in children nearing skeletal maturity should be treated with closed reduction and k-wire fixation.

In the presence of an open fracture, well-established protocols of antibiotic administration, debridement, fracture stabilisation and soft tissue cover should be adhered to.

10.7.4   Complications

Fractures at the base of the first metatarsal may involve the growth plate. Growth arrest here may lead to shortening of the first metatarsal and subsequent deficiency of the medial longitudinal arch. There is little data on the long-term outcome of metatarsal fractures in children.

10.8 Phalangeal Fractures

10.8.1 Epidemiology

Fractures of the phalanges in the paediatric foot are usually caused by a direct trauma from a fallen object or from kicking an object. In younger children they are quite uncommon and the incidence increases with age. About one quarter of these injuries occur in the great toe.

10.8.2 Classification

Phalangeal fractures may be intra- or extra-articular. Those involving the physis can be classified as per the Salter and Harris classification.

10.8.3 Diagnosis

See above.

10.8.4 Treatment, Follow-Up, Complications

The majority of the phalangeal injuries tend to be undisplaced. "Neighbour strapping" to the adjacent uninjured toe, which serves as a splint, is adequate. Malrotation should be corrected. The nail bed of the injured toe should be in the same plane as the others. To avoid maceration when taping, gauze should be placed between the toes. This may be continued for 3–4 weeks or until the child is asymptomatic. During this period it may be unwise for the active child to wear open toed shoes as unintentional contact with an object may be very painful.

Intra-articular injuries involving the proximal phalanx of the great toe include Salter-Harris type III and IV injuries. If the fractures involve more than a third of the joint surface and are displaced, open reduction and internal fixation is indicated. Fixation can be carried out with a K-wire, which is left proud of the skin and then removed after 3 weeks. Leaving such fractures untreated may lead to pain and instability (Fig. 10.4).

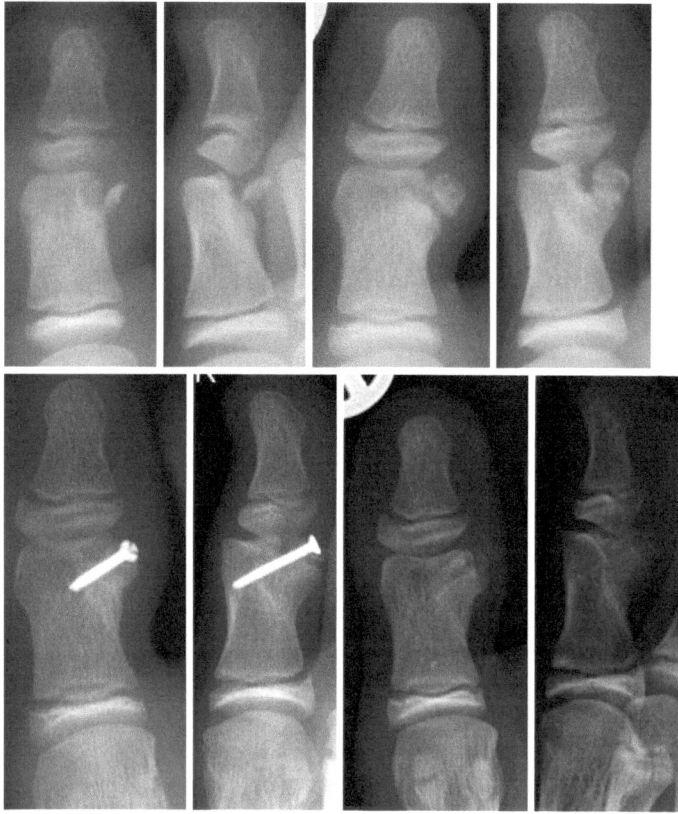

FIGURE 10.4 Intraarticular fracture of the proximal phalanx of the big toe. Despite fracture displacement, the patient was treated conservatively. Two years after the injury, revision surgery was required due to increasing pain and instability. The final outcome was good

10.9   Compartment Syndrome

Compartment syndrome of the foot is uncommon in children but its treatment and operative decompression does not differ to that of the adult. It should be noted that it may occur in the absence of fractures particularly in crush and high-energy injuries. As with compartment syndrome of the limbs, neurovascular compromise is a late finding and should not be relied upon as a diagnostic guide. Compartment pressure monitoring has its place in the assessment of the polytraumatised child with an altered level of consciousness. In a cooperative and awake child, the decision to surgically decompress the foot is made clinically and not based solely on compartment pressure measurements. A massively swollen foot that has been recently involved in high-energy trauma, exhibiting plantar ecchymosis and extensive bruising is in imminent danger of developing compartment syndrome.

Key References

Silas SI, Herzenberg JE, Myerson MS, Sponseller PD. Compartment syndrome of the foot in children. J Bone Joint Surg Am. 1995;77(3):356–61.

Eberl R, Singer G, Schalamon J, Hausbrandt P, Hoellwarth ME. Fractures of the talus – differences between children and adolescents. J Trauma. 2010;68(1):126–30.

Schmidt TL, Weiner DS. Calcaneal fractures in children. An evaluation of the nature of the injury in 56 children. Clin Orthop Relat Res. 1982;(171):150–5. PubMed PMID: 7140063.

Singer G, Cichocki M, Schalamon J, Eberl R, Hollwarth ME. A study of metatarsal fractures in children. J Bone Joint Surg Am. 2008;90(4):772–6.

Mellado JM, Ramos A, Salvadó E, Camins A, Danús M, Saurí A. Accessory ossicles and sesamoid bones of the ankle and foot: imaging findings, clinical significance and differential diagnosis. Eur Radiol. 2003;13 Suppl 6:L164–77. Epub 2003 Aug 6. PubMed PMID: 16440220.

Benson M. Children's orthopaedics and fractures. New York: Springer; 2009.

Chapter 11
Sports Injuries in Children

Panteleimon Chan and Manoj Ramachandran

11.1 Introduction

Anatomical and biomechanical differences compared to adults make children susceptible to a unique spectrum of injuries. These can be acute, in the form of direct or indirect trauma, or chronic overuse injuries, with the failure of specific tissue types. Physeal injuries are common, due to the relative weakness compared with ligaments and ossified bone, and are covered in detail in Chap. 1.

11.2 Strains, Contusions and Sprains

A *strain* is an injury to an area of interface between two tissue types (muscle/tendon, tendon/bone or muscle/bone). *Contusions* are acute injuries to the muscle belly. In comparison, *sprains* are ligamentous injuries.

P. Chan, MBBS, BSc (Hons), MRCS, MRCGP (✉)
Davenport House Surgery, Harpenden, Hertfordshire, UK
e-mail: panteleimon.chan@gmail.com

M. Ramachandran, MBBS(Hons), MRCS, FRCS(Tr&Orth)
Consultant Orthopaedic and Trauma Surgeon,
Paediatric and Young Adult Orthopaedic Unit,
The Royal London and Barts and The London Children's Hospitals,
Barts Health NHS Trust, London, UK

N.A. Aresti et al. (eds.), *Paediatric Orthopaedic Trauma in Clinical Practice*, In Clinical Practice,
DOI 10.1007/978-1-4471-6756-3_11,
© Springer-Verlag London Ltd. 2015

Strains are divided into three grades:

- Grade I – a few fibres are torn, but the surrounding fascia is intact. Clinically, there is swelling, bruising, tenderness, and pain on movement against resistance.
- Grade II – many fibres are torn. There may also be tears of the fascia, partial tears at the musculotendinous junction, and possibly a palpable defect.
- Grade III strains – complete muscle rupture, a palpable defect, and loss of function. Management consists of ice and compression within the first few hours. A short period of rest and immobilization in a lengthened position allows new sarcomere units to fill the gap. This should be followed by passive stretching and then, gentle active mobilisation.

11.3   Myositis Ossificans Circumscripta

This is a relatively uncommon phenomenon whereby new bone is formed within a muscle following a severe contusion from a direct blow. This usually affects the quadriceps and brachialis muscles of young adults and adolescents. The clinical presentation is similar to contusions, with painful swelling and loss of movement. Radiographs demonstrate progressive formation of heterotopic bone from around 3–4 weeks post injury, with a central radiolucent area being surrounded by a more radio-opaque border. This is termed the zonal phenomenon and represents mature ossification around an immature centre. Bone scans may identify this earlier. CT can demonstrate a similar pattern to radiographs, while MRI may not be as specific. Following a period of rest, active mobilization without passive stretching should be started. The side effect of NSAIDs impairing bone formation can be utilized whilst providing analgesic requirements.

11.4   Brachial Plexus Injuries

The causal mechanism for these injuries is usually a direct impact to the shoulder with the neck tilted to the opposite side, such as in rugby or American football.

Brachial plexus injuries can be graded as per Seddon's classification:

- Grade I – neurapraxia, which spontaneously resolves.
- Grade II – axonotmesis usually affecting the upper trunk of the plexus, causing deltoid and/or biceps weakness. Symptoms persist for 4 weeks, with recovery by 6 weeks. Up to 6 months may be required to achieve return to competitive sport.
- Grade III – neurotmesis, where the deficit persists for 1 year.

Symptoms include weakness, burning pain and paraesthesiae. Investigations should include plain radiographs initially to exclude cervical spine or clavicle fractures. An EMG should match the clinical picture. Management is ideally prevention through the use of proper protective safety equipment and technique. Neck stretching and strengthening exercises will also help to guard against injury. Early exploration and repair or reconstruction at 2–4 months for persistent non-resolving deficits or those that are healing in an anatomically inconsistent manner is advocated to maximize the recovery potential.

11.5   Spondylolysis, Spondylolisthesis and Spondylosis

These conditions are associated with chronic hyperextension exercises, such as in gymnastics. Spondylolysis is the term used to describe an anatomic defect of the pars interarticularis, or a "pars defect". They are not present at birth but develop over time. They most commonly occur at the L5/S1 level (Fig. 11.1). Spondylolisthesis is the forward translation of one vertebral body atop the adjacent body, due to posterior element instability. Congenital and isthmic causes are the most common within the paediatric population. Around 15% are associated with a pars interarticularis lesion. The Meyerding classification is based on the severity of the slip:

FIGURE 11.1 Lateral radiograph demonstrating L5/S1 spondylolysis

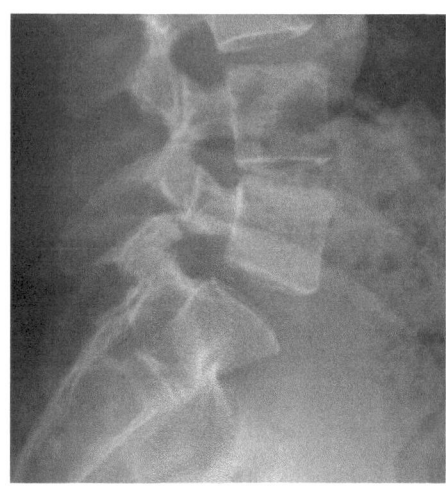

1. Grade I — 0–25% slip.
2. Grade II — 26–50% slip.
3. Grade III — 51–75% slip.
4. Grade IV — 76–99% slip.
5. Grade V — Spondyloptosis, or 100% slip.

The presentation is with lower back pain, which is usually unilateral, and worse with hyperextension or rotation. Examination reveals hyperlordosis, weak abdominal muscles and tenderness that is worst at the belt line. Symptoms are reproduced by extension, particularly unilateral extension when the patient leans back whilst standing on one leg. Pain is worst on the ipsilateral side. There may also be relative hamstring tightness and a pelvic waddling gait. Normal neurology can be expected for pars defects, but with higher grades of spondylolisthesis, signs of compression may be present.

Initial imaging with plain radiographs including AP, standing lateral and both oblique views, can show the pars defect "collar" on Lachapele's "Scotty dog" view. As the athlete may present very early, a technetium 99 bone scan may highlight a defect before radiographic findings. They are also of benefit in differentiating acute lesions needing more aggressive treatment, from chronic lesions. SPECT (single photon emission computed tomography) and CT (computed tomography) add further information to guide treatment.

Management of acute spondylolysis varies, but the consensus involves short periods of bed rest if required, or the utilization of a brace, followed by a generalized fitness program where aggravating activities are avoided. Treatment of chronic lesions is symptomatic. Spondylolisthesis, if less than 50%, may be managed nonoperatively and sport may be allowed, albeit with strong advice regarding potential of further slippage and long term problems. If more than 50%, restriction of activities is recommended and surgery may be considered. For further information, see Chap. 5.

11.6   Shoulder Injuries

11.6.1   Anterior Shoulder Instability

Anterior shoulder instability related to sport is associated with the combination of abduction, external rotation and extension of the joint. The spectrum includes acute dislocations, recurrent subluxations as well as recurrent dislocations. Clinical presentation is with pain, a tender anterior swelling, and "squaring-off" of the shoulder. Examination characteristically demonstrates absence of external rotation whilst the shoulder is dislocated, and must include neurovascular assessment pre-reduction, especially for the axillary and musculocutaneous nerves. Plain radiographs including anteroposterior and Y- or axillary views can confirm or exclude an associated fracture.

Management consists of reduction, immobilization and rehabilitation. Reduction can be done via one of several methods, with aid of muscle relaxants and anaesthesia when available. Care must be taken not to cause traction injury to nerves. Scapular rotation or Stimson's methods are done with the patient prone, whilst the modified Kocher's, double sheet and Hippocratic methods are utilized when supine.

Neurovascular examination and radiographs must be repeated post-reduction to ensure that the humeral head is located and no iatrogenic complications have occurred. Immobilisation to allow for capsular healing should be followed by graded range of movement and muscle strengthening exercises. Return to sport should be delayed for at least 3 months.

Athletes may often have an increased range of movement than normal, particularly those involved in throwing or swimming. This asymptomatic movement may border on subluxation. Recurrent subluxation may also cause these athletes to present with pain mimicking impingement, clicking or neurological symptoms. Recurrent dislocation may have a voluntary element, which may require psychiatric input. Surgical stabilization in voluntary dislocators is more prone to failure, so this must be assessed prior to any operation. Examination of range of movement and stability includes the anterior apprehension test and observing for the sulcus sign. Examination under anaesthesia may also be of diagnostic benefit. Note should be made of the patient's general laxity, e.g. using Beighton's score. Imaging may show a Hill Sachs or Bankart lesion. Operative procedures include the open Bankart procedure, with or without capsular shift, and arthroscopic stabilization.

11.6.2   Proximal Humeral Epiphysiolysis (Little League Shoulder)

Repetitive throwing can cause chronic microtrauma to the proximal humeral epiphysis. Patients present with limitation of activity and localized tenderness on palpation. Widening of the epiphysis can be seen on radiographs. Treatment is symptomatic, with rest until comfort allows return to throwing.

Clavicular and proximal humeral fractures, and acromioclavicular joint injuries are covered in Chap. 2.

11.7   Elbow Injuries

11.7.1   Little League Elbow

Young throwing athletes are susceptible to chronic valgus overloading, resulting in repetitive microtrauma to the medial and lateral structures, varying with the phases involved in the throwing motion and the patient's age. Medial pain results from valgus traction causing medial epicondyle apophysitis, avulsion fractures, medial epicondylitis and ulnar collateral ligament sprains or tears, with increasing skeletal maturity. Laterally, compressive forces acting on the capitellum during cocking and acceleration may lead to avascular necrosis (Panner's disease) or osteochondritis dissecans. Conversely, traction forces in the follow-through phase produce apophysitis of the lateral epicondyle or injury to the radial physis.

Clinical presentation is with elbow pain, predominantly affecting the medial side that impairs the athlete's performance. Radiographs may be normal, or indicate particular age-related pathology. Imaging of the non-affected side together with stress views may be of benefit. MRI may have increased sensitivity, but clinical suspicion must prompt treatment. Management is by resting the elbow from the causal stresses for 4–6 weeks. Following this, a graded return to throwing over a further 4–6 weeks may be started.

11.8   Hip and Pelvic Injuries

11.8.1   Avulsion Fractures and Apophysitis

Avulsion fractures occur rather than strains, particularly at the origins or insertions of muscles around the pelvis or hip. The mechanism may be by indirect trauma or chronic repetitive

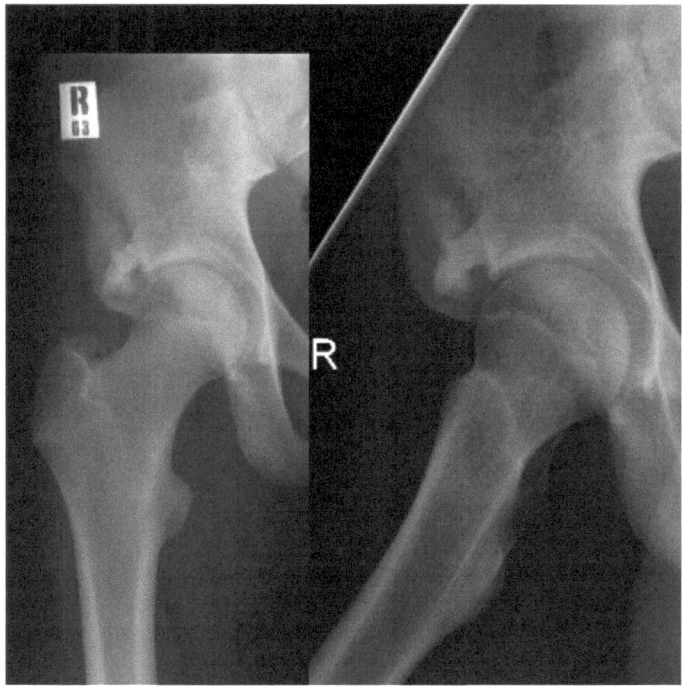

FIGURE 11.2 Chronic pincer changes following an anterior inferior iliac spine avulsion

microtrauma. Areas typically affected include the anterior superior iliac spine (ASIS) due to the pull of sartorius, the anterior inferior iliac spine (AIIS) due to rectus femoris (Fig. 11.2), the ischial apophysis due to the hamstrings, and the lesser trochanter due to iliopsoas. Radiographs help confirm the diagnosis and are useful in follow-up, when the secondary ossification centre can be seen displaced from its anatomical location. Confusion may arise when the secondary ossification centre is not yet visible. Management is usually non-operative, with limitation of muscle usage followed by graded return to sport. Surgical repair is usually reserved for large fragments or resultant loss of function, which is more common at the elbow's medial epicondyle and the knee's tibial tubercule.

There are usually no long-term limitations, unless the resultant healed bone causes secondary impingement.

11.8.2   Iliac Crest Apophysitis

Iliac crest apophysitis usually affects the anterior half of the crest and is caused by pull of the abdominal wall musculature. It is seen in the adolescent runner complaining of persistent hip pain limiting participation. Examination reveals tenderness over the crest and pain on lateral rotation. Management is by modification of activity including avoidance of running for several weeks whilst maintaining fitness through other exercises.

11.8.3   Snapping Hip

Snapping hip is a disorder in which patients experience a snapping sensation in their hips. There are three types: internal, external and intra-articular, based on the site in which a muscle/tendon encounters a bony prominence:

- *Internal snapping:* due to the iliopsoas tendon moving sharply over the femoral head, prominent iliopectinal ridge, exostoses of the lesser trochanter or an iliopsoas bursa. This is the most common form.
- *External snapping:* due to the iliotibial band passing over the greater trochanter.
- *Intra-*articular *snapping:* due to loose bodies in the hip (e.g. synovial chondromatosis) or labral tears.

Patients present with a snapping sensation around their hip joint that may or may not be associated with deep groin pain and tenderness. Clinical examination focuses on recreating the snapping through provocative manoeuvers. External snapping is diagnosed by flexing the hip, with a sudden jolt or snap visible. Pressure over the greater trochanter may eliminate the snapping, confirming the diagnosis. Internal snapping is recreated by moving the hip from a flexed and externally rotated position to an extended and internally rotated one. A more audible snap may well be witnessed.

Snapping hips are common in runners and dancers. Dynamic ultrasonography may aid diagnosis and localisation, identifying thickened tendons. Management is predominantly symptomatic, with the use of analgesia, in particular NSAIDs, whilst abstaining from exacerbating activities. Physiotherapy focuses on stretching and eccentric strengthening exercises. In refractory cases, arthroscopic assessment of any additional intra-articular pathology, together with soft tissue releases, should be considered.

11.8.4   Hip Pointer (Iliac Crest Contusion)

This is caused by direct trauma and is associated with contact sports such as rugby or football. A large haematoma is seen surrounding the iliac wing. Bleeding often occurs into the abductor muscles. Patients are usually managed along RICE principles (rest, ice, compression, elevation), but occasionally benefit from aspiration of the haematoma. Athletes return to sport when comfortable, aided by additional padding.

11.9   Knee

11.9.1   Osteochondritis Dissecans (OCD)

Despite what the name suggests, OCD is not an inflammatory process. It is characterized by separation of hyaline cartilage from the underlying bone. There are two types: a juvenile type that effects children under the age of 12 before the growth plates have fused, and an adult type occurring after fusion. The aetiology of lesions is not fully understood. Repetitive and occult trauma have been implicated, as has idiopathic ischemia.

Lesions most often affect the lateral aspect of the medial femoral condyle. Lateral condyles are affected in 20% of patients, and rarely the patella. Patients present with anterior knee pain, a limp and mechanical symptoms of the joint, including locking and "giving way". This condition is not

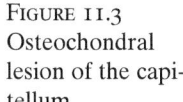

FIGURE 11.3
Osteochondral
lesion of the capi-
tellum

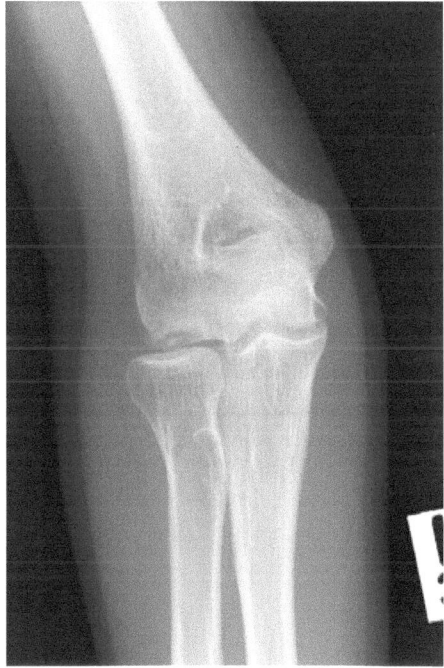

however exclusive to the knee, and may also affect the ankle, hip, elbow (Fig. 11.3) and other joints.

Radiographs, including skyline and tunnel views, demonstrate the defect. MRI scans further define the anatomy and allow assessment of size and stability. Perifocal sclerosis is a negative prognostic indicator. Initial treatment is rest, with surgery reserved for persistent symptoms and for unstable fragments, with fixation or excision of large displaced fragments. Arthroscopy allows direct visualization of the fragment, testing of stability and fixation, drilling or excision.

11.9.2   Apophysitis – Osgood-Schlatter's Disease

Osgood-Schlatter's Disease is a traction apophysitis of the tibial tubercule from repetitive stress exerted by the extensor mechanism. It most often affects adolescent males during a period of rapid growth. Patients will describe focal pain and

FIGURE 11.4 Lateral radiograph showing ossicle formation in Osgood-Schlatter's disease of the knee

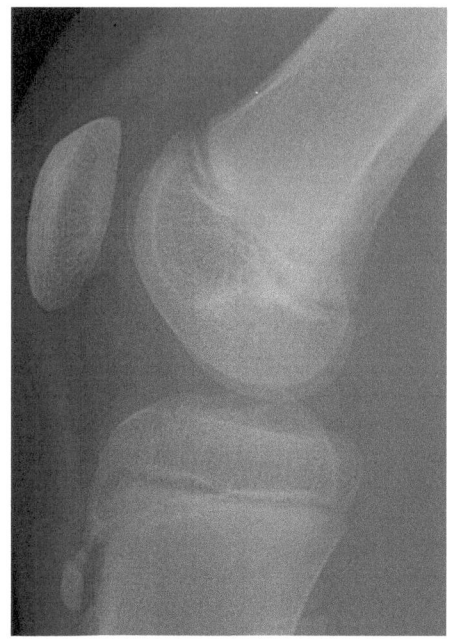

tenderness over the tibial tubercule and there may be an associated bony swelling as well as pain on extension against resistance. Radiographs aid in confirming the diagnosis (Fig. 11.4). Most cases resolve with rest, analgesia and gradation of activity together with eccentric quadriceps strengthening exercises. Surgical excision of the ossicle and tubercleplasty once skeletal maturity has been attained may occasionally be needed for ongoing symptoms.

11.9.3   Tendonitis – Sinding-Larsen-Johansson Syndrome

"Jumper's knee" is an injury at the patellar attachment of the extensor mechanism, due to chronic repetitive stress. As there is no bony abnormality, radiographs are often unremarkable. The condition is self-limiting and management is as per Osgood-Schlatter's disease.

11.9.4   Medial Collateral Ligament Injuries

Medial collateral ligament (MCL) injuries in isolation are a common sporting injury, occurring through the application of valgus stress to the knee whilst the foot is firmly planted on the ground. In the presence of a twisting injury, there may be an associated anterior cruciate ligament (ACL) tear. Examination highlights localized tenderness over the ligament and its origin or insertion. There may be an effusion, which when very large, suggests further pathology.

Valgus stress testing should be performed in 30° of flexion, isolating the superficial MCL. Opening of the medial side when compared to the opposite knee indicates an injury, which is graded as per the amount of displacement (1–4 mm=grade I, 5–9 mm=grade II, >10 mm=grade III). Laxity on valgus stress with a fully extended knee suggests concomitant posteromedial capsule or cruciate injury.

Plain radiographs are commonly normal. Often stress views may be necessary to identify gapping through a physeal (undisplaced Salter-Harris type I) fracture. The Pellegrini-Stieda sign, which is ectopic calcification in the damaged ligament, may be seen in late presentations (Fig. 11.5). MRI can assist in clarifying diagnostic uncertainty.

RICE principles (rest, ice, compression, elevation) are employed immediately after an acute injury. Rehabilitation follows a goal-orientated program, with the use of a hinged knee brace in more severe tears. Maintenance of weight bearing, range of motion, and general fitness help the athlete return to sport earlier, which is possible when they can pass a functional running test. Surgical options in severe (grade III) injuries include repair and reconstruction of the ligament.

11.9.5   Cruciate Ligament Injuries

Anterior cruciate ligament (ACL) injuries in children are similar to adults in terms of mechanism of injury and presentation with clinical signs of a positive anterior draw, Lachman and pivot shift tests. However the injury is more commonly an avulsion of the tibial spine, as the tendon strength often outweighs that of the bone. Radiographs and MRI can non-invasively confirm rupture and fracture, whilst arthroscopy

FIGURE 11.5
Pellegrini-Stieda
sign in chronic
medial collateral
ligament injury

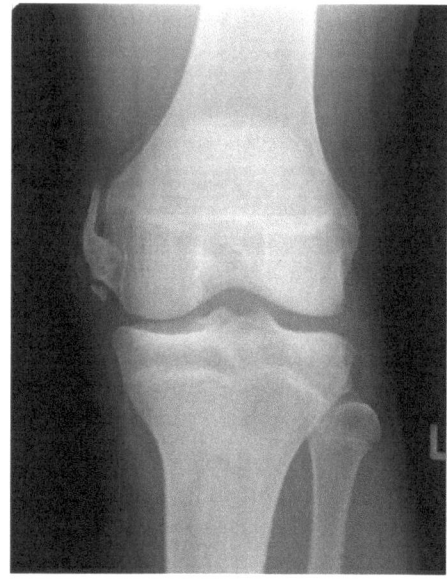

allows direct visualisation. Management depends on the patient's skeletal maturity, aspirations and sporting activities. If the tibial spine has avulsed, reduction with or without fixation is required, which can be done either arthroscopically or open. If the physis is still open, bracing, physiotherapy and modification of participation is utilized, while reconstruction can be performed in elite athletes. Once the physis is closed, reconstruction in the same manner as adults may be performed.

Posterior cruciate ligament injuries are unusual and are usually due to hyperextension. The patient complains of posterior knee pain, a feeling of instability and there may be a haemarthrosis acutely. Radiographs may also show an avulsion fracture. Management is generally non-operative, with consideration for acute reconstruction being reserved for the elite athlete with severe laxity.

11.9.6   Patellar Subluxation/Dislocation

Patellofemoral instability is relatively common, often presenting with acute dislocation. Assessment of associated ligamentous injuries should also accompany patella and extensor mechanism examination, noting patellar position (especially alta), the Q-angle, apprehension sign, and rotational or angular limb deformities. An osteochondral fracture may also be present, and so anteroposterior, lateral, tunnel and skyline view radiographs are needed. These may also reveal a shallow sulcus or bipartite patella. MRI aids assessment of soft tissues and chondral, as well as bony, injuries.

Aspiration of the joint may be required for symptomatic relief of pain. Initial immobilization should be followed by progressive rehabilitation, including isometric exercises to prevent progression of chronic instability. Strengthening of quadriceps, gluteal and tensor fascia lata muscles are all required.

Soft tissue reconstruction may be necessary for refractory instability despite physiotherapy. Procedures to achieve realignment include lateral release, medial VMO (vastus medialis obliquus) reefing, proximal procedures such as tube realignment and/or distal procedures such as Roux-Goldthwaite transfers or tibial tubercule medialisation.

11.9.7   Meniscal Tear

The menisci gradually lose cellularity and vacularity from birth, reaching an adult level at around 10 years of age, making adolescents susceptible to injuries requiring intervention. The mechanism usually involves compression and rotation in flexion, but children are often unable to recall or accurately describe the details of events leading to injury. A full knee examination should be performed to assess for associated ligamentous injuries or instability, as well as to confirm meniscal pathology. Radiographs are useful to exclude osteochondral or physeal fractures. MRI provides non-invasive information on the soft tissues, whilst arthroscopy allows direct visualization and tear stability testing. Stable partial thickness vertical tears, together with small full thickness vertical tears in the more vascular peripheral third as well as short radial tears, may be treated conservatively. Larger vertical tears in the vascular periphery can be repaired. Otherwise, partial or total meniscectomy is required, although preservation of maximal meniscal tissue is advised. There may be an underlying discoid meniscus, which should be addressed with meniscoplasty and/or stabilisation.

11.9.8   Discoid Meniscus

Another cause of paediatric meniscal pathology is the presence of a discoid meniscus. Three types have been described, with complete discoid menisci extending to the tibial spine, whilst incomplete have extra tissue medial to the free end, but not reaching the tibial spine. The final Wrisberg ligament type lacks the posterior meniscal attachment, instead only being attached by the menisco-femoral ligament of Wrisberg. The patient complains of a history of snapping or catching, with palpable clicking. MRI and/or arthroscopy can identify this pathology. If locking and effusion are absent, the knee may be treated non-operatively. Otherwise, meniscoplasty (debulking by partial meniscectomy of the central area) to leave a normal sized intact and stable rim and rim stabilisation in the unstable variant is advised.

11.10   Foot and Ankle

11.10.1   Sever's Disease

This is an apophysitis affecting the calcaneum at the insertion of the Achilles tendon. It is associated with periods of rapid growth and may be confused with tendonitis. The patient presents with heel pain and tenderness. Radiographs show irregular ossification of the apophysis, although this is non-specific. Management is by analgesia, modulation of activity, Achilles tendon stretches, together with a heel cup cushion orthosis to reduce impact loading. Spontaneous resolution is expected with closure of the physis.

11.10.2   Os Trigonum

This is an accessory ossicle just posterior to the talus, of unclear origin. Symptoms of impingement on plantar-flexion, particularly in ballet dancers, or pain from fractures, are the usual reason for presentation. Fractures are treated with initial immobilization and non-weight bearing for 6 weeks, similar to ankle fractures.

Ankle fractures and sprains are covered in Chap. 9.

Key References

Jayakumar P, Barry M, Ramachandran M. Orthopaedic aspects of paediatric non-accidental injury. J Bone Joint Surg Br. 2010;92(2): 189–95.

Soprano JV. Musculoskeletal injuries in the pediatric and adolescent athlete. Curr Sports Med Rep. 2005;4(6):329–34.

Caine D, Caine C, Maffulli N. Incidence and distribution of pediatric sport-related injuries. Clin J Sport Med. 2006;16(6):500–13.

McTimoney CA, Micheli LJ. Current evaluation and management of spondylolysis and spondylolisthesis. Curr Sports Med Rep. 2003;2(1):41–6.

Kocher MS, Waters PM, Micheli LJ. Upper extremity injuries in the paediatric athlete. Sports Med. 2000;30(2):117–35.

Adirim TA, Cheng TL. Overview of injuries in the young athlete. Sports Med. 2003;33(1):75–81.

Chapter 12
Non-accidental Injury

Nick A. Aresti and Mark (J.M.H.) Paterson

12.1   Introduction

Non-accidental injury (NAI) is the preferred term for injury deliberately inflicted on a child as a form of physical child abuse. It may be extended to include injuries occurring as a result of inappropriate or inadequate parenting behaviour. This chapter covers the orthopaedic aspects of such injuries.

NAI is a universal phenomenon although cultural differences and variations in reporting mechanisms in different countries may lead to an underestimation of the problem in some areas.

Most fractures or dislocations caused by NAI occur in young children under the age of 2 years. In particular, fractures under the age of 4 months are very likely to have

N.A. Aresti, MBBS, BSc (Hons), MRCS (✉)
T&O SpR Percivall Pott Rotation,
London, UK
e-mail: email@nickaresti.com

M.(J.M.H.) Paterson, FRCS
Consultant Orthopaedic and Trauma Surgeon,
Paediatric and Young Adult Orthopaedic Unit,
The Royal London and Barts and The London Children's Hospitals,
Barts Health NHS Trust, London, UK

N.A. Aresti et al. (eds.), *Paediatric Orthopaedic Trauma in Clinical Practice*, In Clinical Practice,
DOI 10.1007/978-1-4471-6756-3_12,
© Springer-Verlag London Ltd. 2015

197

been as a result of abuse. Suspicion that a musculoskeletal injury may not have been caused by accidental trauma should be raised in the following circumstances:

12.1.1 Presentation

- Delayed presentation following injury.
- Vague, inconsistent and varying history from carers.
- Inappropriate reactions from parent(s) or carer(s).
- Patient or sibling(s) on a child protection register.

12.1.2 Injury

- Lower limb long bone fracture prior to walking age.
- Multiple fractures, particularly if they are of different ages.
- Soft tissue injuries unrelated to the skeletal injury.

12.1.3 Clinical Assessment

It is essential to document clearly and fully all clinical findings as there is a high chance that these records will be used in a legal context.

The clinical signs of fracture are as seen in "normal" accidental injury; it is important to examine the whole body including the trunk, head and neck in order to pick up injuries that may have occurred at another time. Details of the skeletal injuries seen are given below.

Common non-skeletal manifestations of NAI include:

- Bruises (most common).
- Bite marks.
- Burns.
- Torn tongue frenulum.
- Reduced range of movement.
- Localised swelling.

The mechanism of abuse is predictive of the fracture pattern, therefore details that should be sought include:

- Direct or indirect injuries.
- Isolated or combination of injuries.
- Evidence of types of mechanisms, such as punches, kicks, burns, twisting, shaking or throwing. Examples of features to look out for include: bruises away from bony prominences, multiple bruises, etc.

Evidence of sexual assault may need to be excluded by a paediatrician. If an associated head injury is suspected a full neurological assessment must be performed, together with an ophthalmological examination to exclude retinal haemorrhage.

When the orthopaedic surgeon is the first point of contact with a suspected NAI, the local Child Protection Lead (usually a paediatrician) must be informed so that the appropriate protocol can be initiated. This will include full examination by a paediatrician, and, in the case of associated head injury, by an ophthalmologist, prior to appropriate imaging studies (see below).

12.2   Investigations

Once NAI is suspected it is necessary to perform a radiological skeletal survey to detect occult fractures. There is no place for the so-called "babygram" in infants (a single-plate exposure of the entire infant) as subtle signs of skeletal injury are likely to be missed. Oblique chest views may show rib fractures more clearly, and a CT scan may be indicated to exclude intracranial haemorrhage. The Royal College of Paediatrics and Child Health has released a report on standards of radiological investigations for NAI. These include a standardised series of images that should be taken as part of a skeletal surgery (Table 12.1).

Occasionally radio-isotope bone scanning may help when plain radiographs are equivocal for skeletal injury. They are

TABLE 12.1 The standard child protection skeletal survey for suspected non-accidental injury

Skull

Anterior posterior (AP), lateral, and Towne's view (the latter if clinically indicated)

Skull radiographs should be taken with the skeletal survey even if a CT scan has been or will be performed

Chest

AP including the clavicles

Oblique views of both of the sides of the chest to show ribs ('left and right oblique')

Abdomen

AP of abdomen including the pelvis and hips

Spine

Lateral: this may require separate exposures of the cervical, thoracic and thorocolumbar regions

If the whole spine is not seen in the AP projection on the chest and abdominal radiographs, additional views will be required

AP views of the cervical spine are rarely diagnostic at this age and should only be performed at the discretion of the radiologist

Limbs

AP of both upper arms

AP of both forearms

AP of both femurs

AP of both lower legs

Posteranterior view of hands

Dorsoplantar view of feet

Reprinted from Swinson et al. [4] with permission from Elsevier

TABLE 12.2 Specificity of fracture types for paediatric non-accidental injury

Fractures with high specificity
Metaphyseal fractures
Rib fractures
Scapular fractures
Outer-end clavicle fractures
Fractures of different ages
Vertebral fractures or subluxation
Digital injuries in non-mobile children
Bilateral fractures
Complex skull fractures
Frequent fractures but with low specificity
Mid-clavicular fractures
Simple linear skull fractures
Single long-bone fractures

particularly useful in rib, spinal and diaphyseal fractures, but not as useful for metaphyseal or skull fractures. Biochemical, haematological and genetic investigations should be considered to exclude NAI. These include bone profiles, markers of metabolic disease and parathyroid levels.

12.3   Specific Injuries (Table 12.2)

12.3.1   Skull Fractures

Accidental skull fractures in young children are uncommon. It is unlikely that a young child will sustain a skull fracture in a fall on the head of less than 1 m. In NAI, skull fractures tend

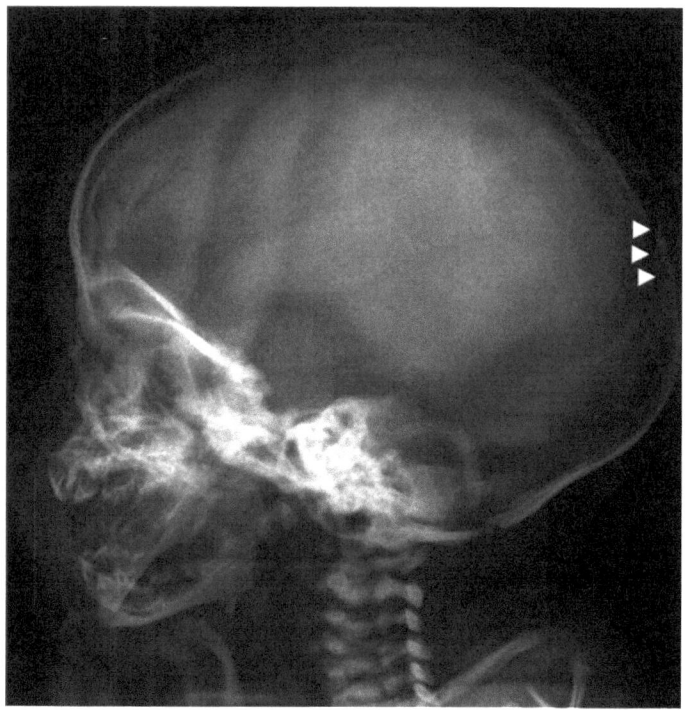

FIGURE 12.1 Linear fracture (*arrowheads*) through the occipital bone of a 2 week old child. This followed a direct blow

to involve more than one bone, and hence to cross suture lines. Suspicion should also be raised in depressed fractures and so-called "growing" fractures, when the fracture gap increases with time (Fig. 12.1).

12.3.2   Rib Fractures

It is rare for rib fractures to occur through accidental trauma in children. Considerable compressive forces are required to cause fractures in the elastic thoracic cage. When they do occur they tend to be multiple and at the posterior angle of the ribs. They are caused by forceful squeezing of the chest by an adult hand (Fig. 12.2).

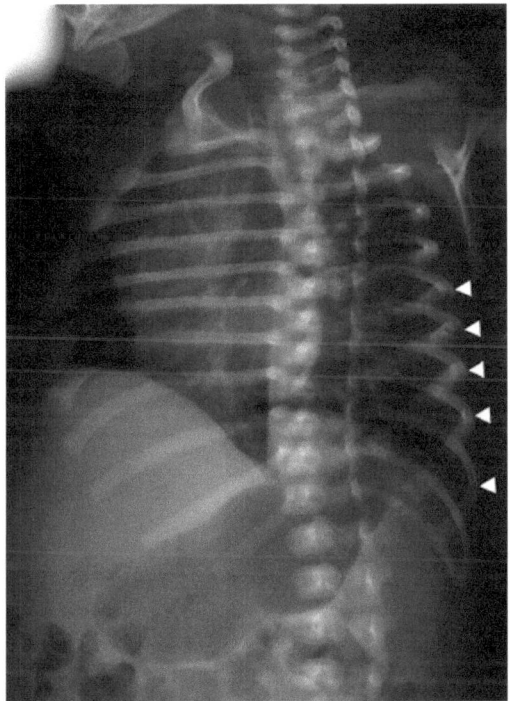

FIGURE 12.2 Rib fractures (*arrowheads*) demonstrated on an oblique radiograph, resulting from a forceful squeeze

12.3.3   Spinal Fractures

These are uncommon, but when they occur, these are indicative of very severe abusive force. They may be flexion or extension injuries, and may or may not have neurological sequelae.

12.3.4   Long Bone Fractures

Diaphyseal fractures may be spiral, oblique or transverse in orientation, depending on the type of abusive force applied. A direct blow or angulation force will result in a transverse fracture, whereas a twisting injury will naturally result in a more spiral configuration. Femoral and tibial fractures in the

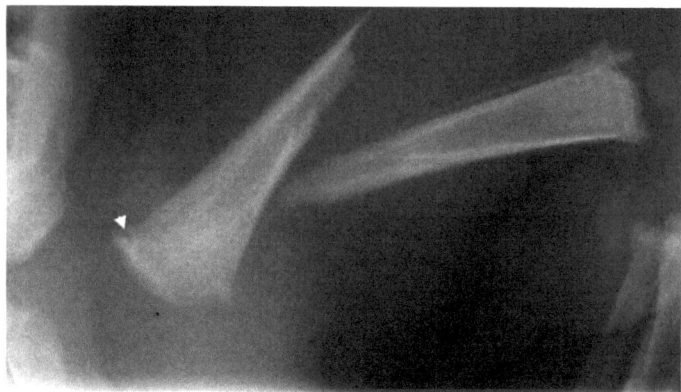

FIGURE 12.3 An oblique diaphyseal fracture with a metaphyseal distal femoral bucket-handle fracture (*arrowhead*) in a 1-year-old child. The mechanism was a twisting injury

non-walking child carry a high risk of being caused by non-accidental means (Fig. 12.3).

The metaphyseal fracture configuration characteristically associated with NAI is the bucket-handle or corner fracture. These can be regarded as avulsion injuries at the margins of joints such as the knee or wrist and are rarely encountered in accidental trauma situations. The alternative names reflect the varying appearance of the fracture, depending on the plane in which it is visualised on radiographs (Fig. 12.4).

The epiphysis may be separated (epiphysiolysis or Salter-Harris I injury); this is sometimes seen at the hip. Particular care is required both at this site and at the elbow in very young infants in whom the ossific nuclei of the respective epiphyses have yet to appear.

12.4   Dating of Fractures

It is not possible to date fracture occurrence with any degree of precision. A rough idea of the timescale involved in the evolution of fracture healing in a young child is given in Table 12.1. The possibility of fracture should not be excluded

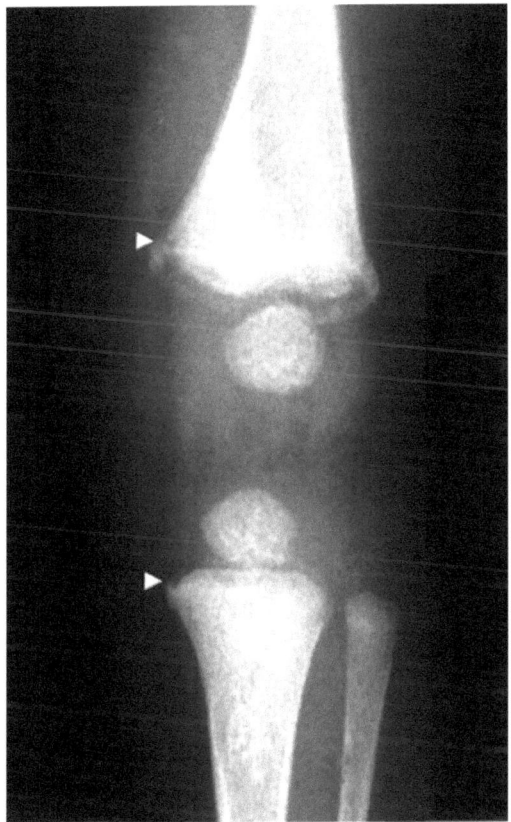

FIGURE 12.4 Bucket handle fractures (*arrowheads*) of the distal femur and proximal tibia following an unknown mechanism of injury in a 14 month old

on the basis of the initial radiographs alone; where suspicion exists, it is important to insist on repeat radiographs 7–10 days later, when the fracture may become apparent.

12.4.1   Periosteal New Bone Formation

It is accepted that rapid acceleration and deceleration forces encountered when a limb is gripped and repeatedly shaken

FIGURE 12.5 Radiograph
showing physiological
new bone formation

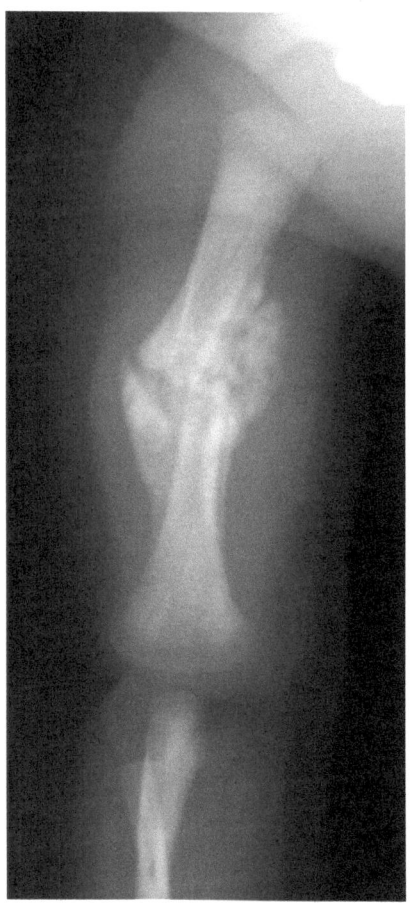

can result in periosteal damage whilst stopping short of
causing actual fracture to the underlying bone. When this
occurs, there may be a florid periosteal reaction, which will
need to be differentiated from that caused by other conditions
(see below) (Fig. 12.5).

12.5   Differential Diagnosis

Differentials of NAI should be considered. Possibilities include:

- Osteopenia of prematurity: very premature infants have osteopenic bones that are more vulnerable to injury.
- Osteogenesis imperfecta (OI): the presence of a family history, blue sclera and Wormian skull bones will help to differentiate in some cases. In mild OI it is uncommon for fractures to occur before walking age. If any uncertainty remains, genetic testing and collagen analysis of skin will make the diagnosis.
- Caffey's disease (idiopathic cortical hyperostosis): this is a rare self-limiting condition characterised by a marked periosteal reaction in long bones in infants but without any other sign of fracture.
- Physiological new bone formation: periosteal new bone is sometimes seen as a normal variant in infants up to the age of 6 months. It does not extend into the metaphyseal region and should therefore not be confused with the extensive reaction seen following non-acidental metaphyseal fractures (Fig. 12.5).

12.6   Fracture Treatment

The treatment of the individual injuries is no different from that of fractures caused by accidental injury. An exception arises in the case of a femoral shaft fracture when an option to treat in traction might be taken as a strategy for keeping the child in hospital under observation whilst the circumstances of injury are investigated.

Provided the injuries are recognised correctly as being non-accidental in origin, and appropriate steps are taken to remove the child from the risk of further injury, the prognosis for each fracture is good. Failure to identify NAI and return of the child to the causative environment will almost inevitably lead to further injury and carries a significant risk of death.

12.7   Summary Points

- High level of suspicion for NAI in long bone fractures in non-walking children.
- Early involvement of relevant child protection agencies.
- Consider possibility of underlying bone disease.

Key References

Jayakumar P, Barry M, Ramachandran M. Orthopaedic aspects of paediatric non-accidental injury. J Bone Joint Surg Br. 2010;92(2): 189–95.

Carty H. Non-accidental injury: a review of the radiology. Eur Radiol. 1997;7:1365–76.

Worlock P, Stower M, Barbor P. Patterns of fractures in accidental and non-accidental injury in children: a comparative study. Br Med J. (Clin Res Ed). 1986; 293(6539):100–102.

Swinson S, Tapp M, Brindley R, et al. An audit of skeletal surveys for suspected non-accidental injury following publication of the British Society of Paediatric Radiology guidelines. Clin Radiol. 2008;63:651–6.

Index

N.A. Aresti et al. (eds.), *Paediatric Orthopaedic Trauma in*   209
Clinical Practice, In Clinical Practice,
DOI 10.1007/978-1-4471-6756-3,
© Springer-Verlag London Ltd. 2015